A Creative Health Communication Framework

This groundbreaking volume offers a theoretical, practical, and evidence-based approach to bridging the gap between service-users, -providers, and -commissioners in order to establish Creative Health as a valued part of healthcare, and a key player in the broader healthcare marketplace.

Offering actionable strategies to strengthen interdisciplinary networks and enrich the Creative Health landscape within modern healthcare systems, the book provides a comprehensive analysis of how economic systems, healthcare philosophy, and societal perceptions shape the uptake and effectiveness of Creative Health services. It outlines the systemic barriers to widespread recognition and identifies how targeted communication can engage both service-users and market forces. Through pragmatic solutions and narrative-based research, chapters present the concept of 'market wellbeing' – a negotiation space that aligns the needs of individuals with healthcare market objectives, fostering stronger connections and sustainability for Creative Health. Ultimately, an entirely novel Creative Health Communication Framework is outlined in the third part of the volume, designed to empower readers with the insights and strategies that can reshape how Creative Health is communicated and valued.

This will be a key volume for scholars, researchers, and postgraduate students in Creative Health, creative arts and expressive therapies, and mental health and health psychology more broadly. Creative Health practitioners should also find this volume of use.

Jane Hearst is a doctor of Creative Health and serves as Midlands Creative Health Associate, National Centre for Creative Health, UK.

Explorations in Mental Health

Understanding Contemporary Diet Culture through the Lens of Lacanian Psychoanalytic Theory
Eating the Lack
Bethany Morris

Learning the Hard Way in Clinical Internships in Social Work and Psychology
Lessons for Safety, Boundary-Setting, and Deepening the Practicum Experience
Susan A. Lord

Mental Healthcare in Brazilian Spiritism: The Aesthetics of Healing
Helmar Kurz

Exploring Creative Wellbeing Frameworks in Context
Nature, Culture, and Sustainable Futures
Edited by Wenche Torrissen and Helga S. Løvoll

A Transdisciplinary Study of Addiction
A New Framework for Drug Policy Reform
Francisco Blancarte Jaber

A Creative Health Communication Framework
Addressing the Compatibility and Marketability of Mental Health and Wellbeing Services
Jane Hearst

For more information about this series, please visit www.routledge.com/Explorations-in-Mental-Health/book-series/EXMH

'Whether you are a researcher, practitioner or student, this book helps to decode the language, practice and power dynamics of the interdisciplinary landscape of Creative Health, its systems and services. Written in the UK context, with global relevance, each chapter makes a thoughtful contribution to further informing the Creative Health sector, specific to mental wellbeing. Furthermore, the 'Creative Health Communication Framework' is a valuable tool, prioritising a user-centred voice and approach, whilst giving confidence to individuals and collaborators driving forward the Creative Health movement. An absolute asset!'

– **Dr Rachel Marsden**, *Research Fellow in Creative-Public Health (NIHR SPHR Transdisciplinary Fellowship), University of Birmingham and Keele University, and Regional Champion (West Midlands) for the Culture, Health and Wellbeing Alliance (CHWA)*

'As CMO of an Integrated Care System (ICS), I value resources that harness the power of Creative Health especially for prevention and early intervention. The framework offered in this book is a vital tool towards that mission, supporting healthcare professionals - both medical and creative - in navigating the complexities of Creative Health commissioning. Elsewhere, chapters help to demystify health and cultural systems, strengthening the synergy needed to advance Creative Health partnerships. It's an excellent resource for anyone committed to enhancing well-being through the arts within our evolving healthcare landscape.'

– **Ananta Dave**, *Chief Medical Officer, Black Country Integrated Care Board, Presidential Lead for retention and wellbeing, Royal College of Psychiatrists, Trustee, Doctors in Distress*

'With Creative Health rapidly becoming a widely recognised health intervention, Hearst's work unpicks the importance of using a universally understood language and active voice to address both terminology, and marketability, for those working in the Creative Health field. This book adds significant and equitable weight to understanding the vital practical, and strategic value, arts and culture contributes to health and social care, and population health promotion.'

– **Amabel Mortimer**, *Creative Health facilitator and educator, Arts, Health and Wellbeing Strategic Lead/Programme Director, University of Gloucestershire, Associate Editor International Journal of Art Therapy*

'Working within governmental public health, I view this book as an essential guide to Creative Health that can broaden the knowledge base of policymakers and public health leaders with clear, market centred language to support the development of governmental priorities and the tools and language needed to justify funding, integrate arts within healthcare strategies and to promote sustainable and populational wide health benefits of the Creative Health field.'

– **Rhys Boyer**, *Senior Public Health Officer, Birmingham City Council Public Health*

A Creative Health Communication Framework

Addressing the Compatibility and Marketability of Mental Health and Wellbeing Services

Jane Hearst

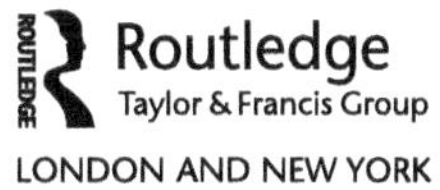

LONDON AND NEW YORK

First published 2025
by Routledge
4 Park Square, Milton Park, Abingdon, Oxon OX14 4RN

and by Routledge
605 Third Avenue, New York, NY 10158

Routledge is an imprint of the Taylor & Francis Group, an informa business

© 2025 Jane Hearst

The right of Jane Hearst to be identified as author of this work has been asserted in accordance with sections 77 and 78 of the Copyright, Designs and Patents Act 1988.

All rights reserved. No part of this book may be reprinted or reproduced or utilised in any form or by any electronic, mechanical, or other means, now known or hereafter invented, including photocopying and recording, or in any information storage or retrieval system, without permission in writing from the publishers.

Trademark notice: Product or corporate names may be trademarks or registered trademarks, and are used only for identification and explanation without intent to infringe.

British Library Cataloguing-in-Publication Data
A catalogue record for this book is available from the British Library

ISBN: 978-1-032-71729-6 (hbk)
ISBN: 978-1-032-72979-4 (pbk)
ISBN: 978-1-003-42331-7 (ebk)

DOI: 10.4324/9781003423317

Typeset in Sabon
by SPi Technologies India Pvt Ltd (Straive)

Contents

Introduction

'The next big thing is the one that makes the last big thing usable'

– Blake Ross

Creativity and the arts have always been closely connected to different aspects of our health and wellbeing. In recent years, this creativity has been more formally labelled, recognised, and advocated for, across the globe, via the Creative Health movement. In the last decade, we have seen a dramatic growth in the evidence base for Creative Health provisions, along with increased political support, the early development of conducive systems, and an upsurge of interest in producing Creative Health strategies within health and social systems. But, until Creative Health can be discussed in clearer terms, its actualisation may be hindered by a lack of popular awareness and the historical bias towards medicine and scientific evidence hierarchies. That is where this book offers a valuable contribution.

What Is Creative Health?

According to the National Centre for Creative Health (NCCH), 'Creative Health' is a term that can be used to describe both a type of activity – which involves arts, culture, heritage, or creativity of any kind – and an approach to healthcare – one which is focused on new possibilities and innovative ways of working (APPG on Arts Health and Wellbeing & NCCH, 2023).

Unpicking this further, I would suggest there are five key areas of Creative Health *activity*. I make these distinctions based on what each activity aims to support: 1) physical health; 2) mental health; 3) wellbeing; 4) health promotion; 5) health-related research. Creative Health activities focusing on physical conditions include services such as singing for lung health or dance-based physiotherapy. These are targeted interventions that can prevent or reduce the symptoms of various physical illnesses and impairments. Similarly, Mental Health activities respond to recognised conditions. For example, NICE recommends that arts therapies are considered for everyone

DOI: 10.4324/9781003423317-1

who has psychosis or schizophrenia (National Institute for Health and Care Excellence, 2014). Wellbeing, on the other hand, is something that extends beyond the medical definition of a mental condition. Activities that support wellbeing are often community based. They respond to issues such as social isolation and health inequalities, or provide a space for improved mood, self-awareness, and playfulness. This often takes place in the form of participatory arts or other creative activities such as community cooking, gardening, or urban design. Health promotion activities use creativity to improve knowledge and behaviour in the population. A good example of this is using museum exhibitions to improve awareness of health conditions. Finally, Creative Health can appear in research activity via the use of unique – and often artistic – research methods, such as Lego serious play, labyrinth making, or digital storytelling.

In regard to Creative Health *approaches*, this is also varied. One example includes the use of local community assets as a way of maintaining capacity in healthcare. Another great example is communicating in non-verbal/non-literal ways of knowing – like using the arts to better understand the experiences of people with dementia. A core value of the Creative Health movement is the inclusion of Lived Experience Experts. For this reason, working equitably with service-users to co-design health solutions may also be considered a Creative Health approach – with or without the use of creative activities as power-levelling facilitators. Likewise, creative responses to health psychology are important for quality health promotion. Some great examples of this include decorating stairs to reduce reliance on lifts/escalators, or putting art in hospitals to increase recovery time and reduce pain. Finally, cultural change in healthcare is a big element of the Creative Health approach. In practice, this can include exercises such as using creative wellbeing activities with staff as a catalyst for more creative, person-centred responses to patient care.

What Does This Book Have to Offer the Creative Health Movement?

With the term 'Creative Health' covering such an expansive range of activity and approaches, it becomes increasingly important that Creative Health researchers, practitioners, and advocates can effectively communicate their unique role and impact within this movement. This book supports communication around mental health and wellbeing services – a type of health which I believe to be more difficult to communicate about within capitalist and/or science-informed marketplaces, compared to physical health provisions.

Communicating the role and impact of creativity on physical health needs is easier, as our healthcare systems have pre-designed labels and criteria for these needs. For example, in the UK, the Department of Health and Social Care has a 'Major Conditions Strategy,' which seeks to reduce hospital demand in six key areas. The NHS has the 'Core20PLUS5' target population strategy, which seeks to reduce health inequality. Moreover, at the level of Integrated Care Boards (ICBs) stakeholders respond to targets set in their Joint Forward Plans. If using categories like these, stakeholder can assign measurable outputs and goals, and different research methods can be prioritised based on the type of data being collected in these outputs. Whilst there are also 'wicked issues' within physical health, which are less easy to quantify and respond to, Creative Health services working in these areas are no more disadvantaged than other provisions working in this messier landscape.

The domain of mental health and wellbeing, on the other hand, is an ever-changing landscape. People's definitions and conceptualisations of mental health and wellbeing differ between systems, cultures, communities, and timelines. Even when a vague definition is shared across stakeholders and collaborators, it can be difficult to attain quantifiable evidence. Perspectives differ on what the relationship is between a defined health need and the proposed 'ideal' outcome.

This book explores some of the key power dynamics, historical conceptualisations, health cultures, public needs, and systematic limitations that shaped the development of the Creative Health Communication Framework and promoted the importance of its creation. Through this exploration, I present pragmatic and cutting-edge options for conducting quality, person-centred Creative Health research, paying close attention to how research and practice are shaped by the barriers of a market system and service-users' unique lifeworlds. I then describe the Creative Health Communication Framework in detail, showcasing real stories from members of the public and Creative Health exemplars from across the cultural and health industries.

Who Is This Book for?

This book is primarily targeted towards readers who are working in Creative Health or with Creative Health collaborators. My exploration of theory will be particularly useful to researchers and practitioners in the field. I hope that this increased sophistication of research, communication, and design will have rippling impacts, improving the accessibility and compatibility of services to those who use them. I consider commissioning bodies to be a secondary beneficiary of this book, as improved precision in promotional communication will improve the quality of the services they fund. I hope that, thanks to this, commissioning bodies – whether public, private, or charitable – can feel more confident in the value of Creative Health and, therefore, funding in this sector can increase.

The framework will be particularly useful for creative practitioners who work outside of traditional healthcare systems and structures, as it helps to communicate with a precision that is not compulsory in the cultural industries. This reflects my experience of working with grassroots Creative Health providers, as opposed to accredited Creative Arts Therapists. I approach artistic promotion from point zero, assuming no particular prior knowledge of the researcher or provider above another. Consequently, different aspects of the framework will prove more helpful to different readers, depending on their personal background.

My work is embedded within a UK context, but there are many elements of it that can prompt discussions that are relevant to other countries. The UK system is world-leading, despite the limitations imposed on it, making it a great exemplar to unravel. Moreover, by limiting examples to a single country, I have been able to demonstrate the ripple effects of the multiple, overlapping systems that influence the power dynamics of a marketplace. It should be noted, however, that countries where healthcare systems are less developed may not face the same opportunities and challenges.

Since the language used within the framework was developed around a user-centred model of wellbeing, readers can become pioneers in user-centred healthcare. Through this, I hope that creative, medical, and community providers, alike, may use this de-pathologised model in their own work. This would allow for more cohesive mental health and social care systems, which are collaborative, equitable, and user-centred, discussing mental health in terms that resonate most meaningfully to the patients and participants they serve.

Key Terminology in This Book

The term **'Creative Health'** was popularised by the APPG on Arts Health and Wellbeing's Creative Health Inquiry Report in 2017. It is a term that is still in its infancy and is not yet widely recognised within the health and care systems. The phrase builds upon terms such as 'arts-in-health,' but expands past the limitations of these terms to celebrate creativity in its widest definition. I will largely be referring to artistic contexts throughout this book; however, my framework can be applied to much broader contexts – even those which do not centre creativity.

My observation is that '**arts-*for*-health**' is typically used to describe services where the arts practitioner is central to the delivery of care, and where they design specifically with the intention of aiding the health or wellbeing of their service-user. This differentiates from '**arts-*in*-health**,' where any type of artistic input is included – such as medical provisions that use the arts only for marketing purposes. Whilst I do not use these terms within this book, it is important to note that I am primarily concerned with the former.

Where I refer to a '**Creative Health service**', this is inclusive of all artforms and creative activities that have the intention or scope of supporting mental health and wellbeing. This includes less conventional therapeutic services, such as sandplay, digital storytelling, zine making, and tattooing, as well as more traditional art forms, such as painting, singing, and dancing. Whilst

I prioritise artists in my examples, other Creative Health activities can include gardening, reading, heritage, and play-based activity.

I have been mindful in prioritising '**mental wellbeing**' over discussions of '**mental health**'. Mental wellbeing is distinct from mental health, as the latter appears most frequently within medical literature where it has often been defined as the absence or presence of acute illnesses of the mind. Mental wellbeing, on the other hand, embraces a eudaemonic approach to psychological measurement, whereby joy and self-actualisation denote a lifestyle that goes beyond simply surviving. By designing around a broader variety of experiences of the mind – from short-term negative emotions to longer-lasting negative wellbeing, and through to clinically significant mental ill-health – I acknowledge the relationship between these states and can provide a language framework to professionals working anywhere along the continuum. Moreover, I recognise the interdependent relationship between physical, mental, and social health (World Health Organisation, 1946). Consequently, the framework I have constructed can be used, both, by service-providers who have designed around specific wellbeing agendas and those who wish to communicate the indirect wellbeing benefits of other provisions.

I define '**promotional communication**' as any interaction between a researcher or service-provider and their service-users, participants, readers, or funders, whereby an opportunity exists to clarify their role and the strengths of Creative Health. This promotion is not, therefore, restricted to marketing material. This is an important distinction, as my goal is to investigate and respond to underdiscussed aspects of the service-user experience. By bringing attention to weaknesses in communication, readers are able to respond to them better pre-, during, and post-engagement with an artistic provision. Within this, I advocate for clear communication about a service's limitations and scope, so that service-users are empowered to manage their expectations and make smart market decisions. I demonstrate how service promotion can be used to increase the mental health literacy of the public and how this can shape their ability to engage with multiple wellbeing services, which specialise in different but complimentary aspects of wellbeing. The framework also provides measures and strategies that can guide researchers and service-providers in the way they *design* their projects and provisions. Through this, I intend to aid Creative Health specialists in making their work more transparent and fundable; ensuring that they can reach the right service-users and demonstrate the place for their service within a collaborative wellbeing market.

I made the choice to investigate '**market value**,' as opposed to the '**moral**' or '**aesthetic**' values of the arts. This choice centres my inquiry within market barriers, paying recognition to that which shapes a service-user's ability to access care. I maintain that a service can hold high moral value and low market value at the same time, and it is only by directing the attention of readers to one specific type of value acquisition that my framework can be appropriately discussed, critiqued, and developed in relation to our current market.

In this book, I define market value as a negotiated output that seeks, both, to benefit a service-user and strategically survive within a philosophically biased environment. Within many market systems, like that of the UK, services are not prioritised based on their moral value to society or the individual, but on their ability to directly develop profit or to supply enough social capital to enhance an individual's engagement within the economy in years to come. Within this system, provisions are talked about in terms of limited financial resources and the services that will be lost if an arts provision is prioritised for funding. I argue, therefore, that being able to articulate the unique mental wellbeing benefits of a Creative Health service in market terms significantly improves the ability for artistic service-providers to successfully advocate for the funding of their provisions. This is true because public, private, and individual funders, alike, are all interested in ensuring value for money within their financial exchange.

Importantly, Creative Health is not limited to services within a marketplace. Everyday engagement with creativity has been shown to significantly improve the quality and length of people's lives (Mansfield et al., 2024; Wright, 2022). However, since the purpose of my framework is to support the compatibility and promotion of fundable provisions, this book will almost exclusively discuss Creative Health in terms of services.

One of my secondary goals for the language framework is to support the accessibility of funding for Creative Health services. However, my primary goal remains to assist service-providers in *attracting users* towards their services, whilst maintaining service-user safeguarding and the compatibility. Consequently, I focus on promotional communication *to* service-users. By increasing public awareness and advocacy for arts services, my hope is that the pressure for public funders and private sponsors to engage in support will increase and the success rate of Creative Health services can naturally rise. To achieve this, service-providers must be able to speak to users on their own terms, paying respect to their ideals and perspectives, and enhancing their sense of trust through transparent and clear communication.

Due to my interest in how the market affects the success of Creative Health provisions (both financially and in terms of user satisfaction), this book might be considered to hold a business-informed epistemology. Importantly, however, I refer to other epistemological features, such as phenomenology, in my chapter on research methodology. I argue that these pre-existing ways of thinking are implicitly shaped by the market, and that my application of business frameworks is used as a mechanism to make those implicit influences explicit. By demonstrating the persistent effect of markets on the everyday functioning of our health and cultural systems, I aim to provide a discussion ground in which traditional health providers and Creative Health professionals, alike, can discuss the provision of care and unite their understandings.

Finally, the breadth of activity that falls within the Creative Health umbrella means that it would be unjust to consider it a single industry. Rather, Creative Health is a multi-sectoral and interdisciplinary landscape, with messiness at its core. From this messiness comes innovation, adaptability, and a sense of humanity, which is why it is important for me to acknowledge. For this reason, I refer to Creative Health activity as both '**industry**' and '**movement.**' This terminology seeks to honour the vast number of stakeholders who are collaboratively progressing the values and visibility of Creative Health, both at national and international scales.

References

APPG on Arts Health and Wellbeing and NCCH (2023) *Creative Health Review: How Policy Can Embrace Creative Health*. London: National Centre for Creative Health and All Party Parliamentary Group on Arts Health and Wellbeing.

Mansfield, L. et al. (2024) Understanding everyday creativity: A framework drawn from a qualitative evidence review of home-based arts. *Annals of Leisure Research*, 27(1), pp. 55–86.

National Institute for Health and Care Excellence (2014) *Psychosis and schizophrenia in adults: Prevention and management*. London: NICE.

World Health Organisation (1946) *Preamble to the Constitution of WHO as adopted by the International Health Conference*.

Wright, J. (2022) *Research Digest: Everyday Creativity*. Leeds: Centre for Cultural Value.

Part 1

Navigating the Existing Market

Chapter 1

The Story That Prompted a Creative Health Communication Framework

Let me tell you a story. A story about Amber. Amber is an intelligent young woman, with a strong will and a curious mind. She loves to reflect, so she has collected mementos throughout her life. But, unfortunately for Amber, some things are not worth remembering.

In 2016, when Amber's family found out about the sexual assault she endured as a teenager, Amber could no longer choose which memories to hold on to. Whilst her family was consumed with rage, focused on notions of justice and revenge, Amber was quietly breaking down under the trauma of her memories and their social interpretations. She felt like an outsider to her own life – everybody loudly declaring their opinion about her assault, but nobody asking what actually happened or how she felt (Figure 1.1).

It is clear from this story that Amber could have benefitted from formal wellbeing support. Yet, when Amber approached the National Healthcare

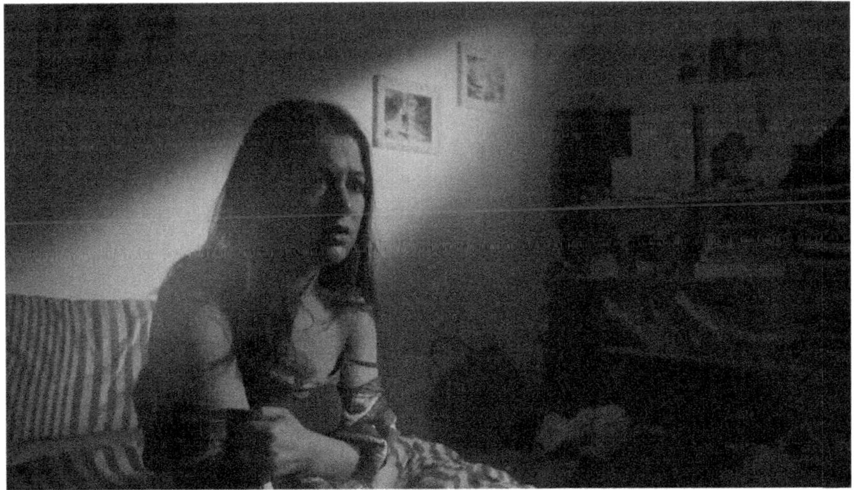

Figure 1.1 Amber sits on a bed, her clothing out of place, her face forlorn.

DOI: 10.4324/9781003423317-3

Service (NHS) in the UK, she was told she may have to wait up to 3 years before she would have access to publicly-funded counselling. As she started to feel like she was losing grip of her reasons to live, Amber knew she couldn't wait that long.

I have started with this story as it sets the scene for what will be explored in this book. Namely, it demonstrates how the weaknesses of a system can negatively impact the wellbeing of an individual who relies on that system. In this case, Amber was affected by the lengthy waiting lists for mental healthcare which have become commonplace in the UK. These waiting lists point towards a bigger problem plaguing the NHS; the fact that there is now more demand for mental health services than there are providers available to deliver care (Baker, Canvin and Berzins, 2019; NHS England and NHS Improvement, 2020). Specifically, it has been estimated that '75% of people with mental health problems in England may not get access to the treatment they need' (Davies and Bucur, 2021, p. S317) and 'policy documents show there [was] an estimated need for more than 6,000 more mental health clinical support staff [between 2021 and 2024]' (Palmer et al., 2021, p. 3).

Whilst these figures are UK-specific, they point to a mental health crisis that is being experienced globally. The World Health Organization explains that mental disorders are the leading global cause of disability worldwide (2021) and the third leading cause of overall disease burden within the European region (2018). In 2022, a team of 41 researchers confirmed that 'mental disorders remained among the top ten leading causes of burden worldwide, with no evidence of global reduction in the burden [across their 29-year dataset]' (GBD Mental Disorders Collaborators, 2022, p. 137). They comment that 'to reduce the burden of mental disorders, coordinated delivery of effective prevention and treatment programmes by governments and the global health community is imperative' (p. 137).

One way of addressing this problem is by diversifying the type of service-providers that can contribute to the delivery of mental health and wellbeing care, such as Creative Health practitioners. This is the first motivation that informs the creation of this book. My logic is that the more we can support Creative Health entrepreneurs to succeed, both, in their service development and promotional communication, the more likely it is that we can increase the number of mental health services available and improve the speed at which service-users can access support.

However, bringing artists into historically medical healthcare systems is not simple. Medical treatments typically respond to patterns that take place in a physical body. They seek predictable outcomes based on non-sentient aspects of human biology. These biological measures can be studied with precision to reduce adverse effects and to maximise the efficiency of treatments, resulting in limited but precise solutions to mental health. Artistic treatments, on the other hand, often respond to wellbeing phenomena that have been uniquely moulded by a sentient mind. These phenomena are impacted by social discourses, culture, politics, physical and emotional environments, physiological sensations, personality types, family dynamics, systematic power relations, popular media, education, philosophy, physical health, neurological processing, communication styles, work pressures, love, interpersonal connection, and so much more. These phenomena are ever-evolving and interact in complex, irregular ways. Consequently, at this side of the mental health continuum, two people faced with relatively similar hardships can hold completely different perspectives and/or experiences of wellbeing. As a result, they require bespoke artistic solutions.

This places Creative Health researchers and service-providers at odds with the current healthcare system, as the established philosophies and procedures can be antipathetic. At the heart of medical procedures, however, are ethics relating to safeguarding, minimising risk, and ensuring valuable returns for taxpayers'/patients' money. I believe that these are values that *should* be embedded into Creative Health services as well. It is for this reason, that I argue there may be a mis-conceptualisation of Creative Health services, by both medical and artistic practitioners alike...

Take a look at academic literature or access professional discourse via a Creative Health event, and it will not take long before you encounter rhetoric about the conflict between scientific precision and artistic flexibility. Conversely, I believe that elements of *both* precision and flexibility must exist in conjunction with one another for Creative Health services to thrive. Specifically, the arts speak well to the conscious and evolving aspects of wellbeing, as they are adaptable. They often reposition the 'patient' into the position of 'knowledge-specialist' (regarding their lived experience or life narrative), and use the arts simply as a tool at their disposal. But, like medical solutions, artistic tools *can* be used more or less effectively, depending on the compatibility of an art-from or facilitator and based on the service-user's mental health literacy. For this reason, precision is an important ethical decision when evaluating the *compatibility* of a Creative Health service, whereas flexibility is important in the *application* of artistic tools, when applied to an individual's unique context.

Without acknowledging this distinction, on where both precision and flexibility belong in the therapeutic arts process, artistic researchers and practitioners may be tempted to communicate to medical peers via the stable truths of their service – such as target demographic, environmental context, or the education of practitioners – even when the key to their success lies in their philosophical approach or intended outcomes. By linking these promotional choices back to their impact on potential service-users, like Amber, I demonstrate how this may negatively impact the success of Creative Health services within a marketplace.

Existing Frames of Promotion

Based on my research, I observe that it is common for artistic provisions to be promoted via their target demographic, particularly when the focus is on vulnerable groups such as young people or the elderly. Amber was 17-years old when she was assaulted and she was 22-years old at the time of experiencing her mental health crisis. She would have fit, therefore, into the categorisation of 'young person' or 'young adult'. Moreover, it would be the vulnerability associated with this aspect of her identity that contributed to her experience of assault. However, I challenge whether this is enough to make a youth-focused provision compatible to her needs. Arguably, there are safeguarding and disclosure concerns related to whether Amber would have felt comfortable to share this information in a group setting and whether the voices of young people were the type that could help her to make sense of her circumstance.

Other ways that research literature promotes provisions include the setting in which they are delivered, such as arts in hospitals or arts in care homes. Amber was not residing within a specific health-related centre at the time of her mental health crisis, which would have isolated her from setting-specific provisions.

Another prominent feature of promotion within research literature is the type of specialism that is held by a service-provider, such as certified art, dance, or music therapists, or participatory arts practitioners from more diverse artistic pathways. Amber could have received care from any number of specialists, which might suggest that choosing a service based purely from the job titles of practitioners was not the most optimal way for her to assess which of these services was right for her.

Outside of the research environment, within the Creative Health market, my observation is that provisions are often promoted for their broad wellbeing benefit, with little information about the who, how's, or what's of the provision. For example, a practitioner who currently uses music for therapeutic purposes within Leicester, promotes her Gong Baths by saying 'Allow yourself to immerse in the healing vibrations of sound' (Kozera, 2022, para. 1), but they do not follow this up with any information about what type of health or wellbeing concerns this music is able to heal. Other provisions are clearer about the type of wellbeing they support, but do not indicate what kind of person or wellbeing context this support is particularly useful for. For example, the public museums and galleries in Leicester promote that 'Museums can be good places to make you feel happy; they give you the space to discover what you like and how you feel as you walk around' (Leicester Museum & Galleries, 2022, para. 1).

If we compare these examples to physical health provisions, surgery may be a great solution for some physical health issues, yet we would not expect it to be the go-to response for every ailment we experience. Accordingly, without context of what a provider defines as healing, and what aspect of wellbeing this contributes to, service-users risk getting lost within the Creative Health landscape or they could find themselves involved with a misaligned service.

If we take these two promotional examples from Leicester as an illustration, we can see that Amber could theoretically have benefitted from either of these services. She was 1) searching for healing and 2) wanted to better understand how she was feeling. But from these descriptions alone, it is unclear whether they can meet her specific needs relating to *trauma* and *relational overwhelm*. This introduces a second problem with the existing market: that promotional material does not communicate clearly enough about what the unique benefits are of different services.

Since Amber's experience back in 2016, social prescribing has been introduced into the UK's healthcare system to help members of the public to access social provisions, such as Creative Health services, more easily. Here, patients who are struggling with their mental health can be directed by their General Practitioner (GP) towards a Social Prescriber who is able to recommend a social provision that can best aid them in their healing or uplift their wellbeing. Social Prescribers – otherwise known as Link Workers or Care Co-ordinators – rely on the promotional material of service-providers and their research partners to allocate suitable provisions to each of their clients.

It is my conviction that the benefits of Creative Health services need to be more clearly articulated to both Social Prescribers and service-users, so that this allocation of support can better fit with service-user needs. This notion is supported by recent evidence. Namely, despite a wealth of literature indicating that the arts can have tremendous effects on the way that people feel, connect, understand themselves, and develop resilience, a recent systematic review on social prescribing in the UK showed that social provisions are failing to demonstrate improved mental health results or provide evidence of their cost effectiveness (Kiely et al., 2022). I hypothesise that this is not an indication that Creative Health research findings are wrong but that, when implemented via social prescribing, there is not enough information to pair the right users with the right projects, or to hold these projects to a sustainable standard of delivery.

There is a crucial reason why I hold this to be true, and it is not something that I could have gathered through literature alone. That is, that Amber's story is, in fact, my own. I was once the individual in need of a support service and, whilst I am a strong advocate of the power of the arts to improve mental health and wellbeing, I know first-hand that the *type* of arts service that is accessed is a vital piece of the mental health puzzle.

To illustrate, one of the services I accessed during my time of need was an artistic mindfulness class where we were encouraged to observe and play with tactically interesting objects, to soak in creative joy, and harness a sense of being present. This service appeared to have a positive impact on other participants within the session, to whom this way of thinking was foreign, but my neurodivergent brain already had no problem in noticing the quirky details of the everyday and it engaged with daydreaming so often that it did not share the temporal concerns of others.

The service was incompatible to my needs. Yet, because there was a lack of precision within the promotional language of how this service could be helpful to certain people's wellbeing, the fact that it had not helped *my* specific type of wellbeing left me feeling more hopeless than ever. These interactions caused me to believe that either I was the problem or that my issues had eroded so much of my mind that I was no longer capable of being helped. The more depressed and anxious I felt, the less energy or motivation I had to engage in other provisions and the more at risk I became of being lost within the system during a moment of serious decline.

The Importance of Service-User Voice

My personal experience motivated another feature of this book: co-creation with service-users. I believe that the detailed and personalised reflections of potential service-users offer service-providers the clearest understanding of what they are missing from their service design and/or promotional communication and how they can improve this.

My experience, alone, has offered me a tremendous degree of knowledge. As an individual that struggled with significant mental health difficulties at the time, I recall the feeling of being underprioritised by my primary care providers due to the large waiting lists and a comment that my sexual assault did not qualify me to be classified as acutely in need. I can explain in great detail why a youth focused, group programme would not have been the place to share my story of assault, no matter how much my youth-related naivety and emotional regulation had made me vulnerable to the incident. I can resonate with the feelings of hopelessness associated with the idea of only being able to access support at the point of hospitalisation for acute mental health needs, rather than the moment I identified them as a problem. I can remember the way that specialist job descriptions went over my head and the stress that was caused by the idea of getting this wrong. I can see why oversimplified statements of wellbeing within promotional material can make the search for support feel like a minefield and recognise the feeling of despair that follows engagement with the wrong service.

I wish that there had been services that told me in clear terms what the scope of their support was. I could have benefited from them making me aware of my co-existing wellbeing needs, so that I could more quickly identify the right services for me. Finally, I know that when the right Creative Health service is accessed, our mental health can transform at a tremendous speed and reach new heights of joy, self-awareness, and self-advocacy. It is because of this that I am convinced that my transformation was something I could not have achieved through traditional, non-arts-based provisions alone.

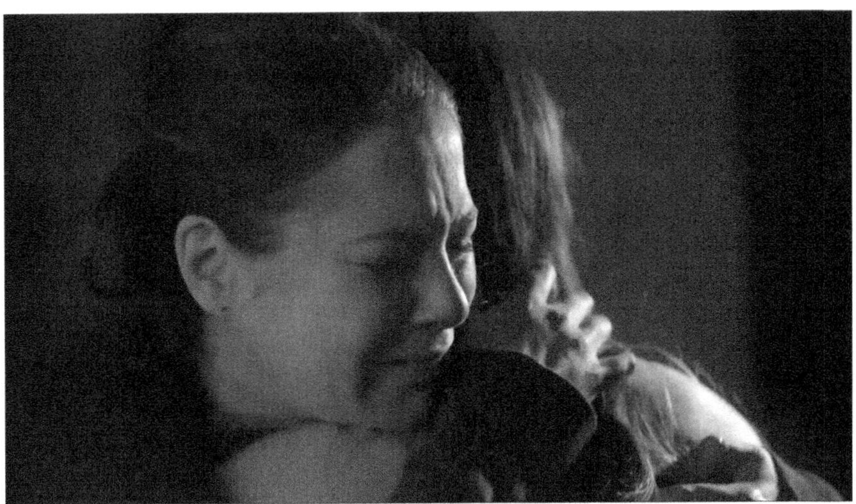

Figure 1.2 Still from *The Past Whispers*; two versions of Amber share a consoling hug.

My story had a happy ending, but this was purely down to luck. Once I had already given up on finding a service that could help me, I was professionally commissioned by Channel 4, Random Acts, to create a short film about my experience (*The Past Whispers*, 2018). It was the act of working with a team of creatives to turn my complex experience into a three-minute story, featuring the character of Amber, that helped me to rewrite my internal narrative about what had happened.

By visually depicting the me of 2016 going back in time to the day of my assault and watching her comfort her younger self (Figure 1.2), I was able to change my perspective of how responsible I was for this happening to me. The film appeared in cinemas, drawing the attention of my friends and family, and this acted as a vehicle to share my experience through an empathy-inducing medium. It saved me from having to verbally repeat the same complex and triggering details to each of the individuals in the audience. Adding to this, I was invited to Directors' Q&A sessions where I was treated as the expert of my own experience. This allowed me to grow confidence in my own voice and use it to help others who had experienced abuse like my own. Using film as a communicative device helped me to take the evolved identity I had created for myself and reintegrate it within the community that I loved. This, in turn, meant that the chances of my new-found identity surviving social discourse, influence, and routine were much easier to actualise.

The reason it is important for me to share some of the intricacies of this filmmaking journey is that it demonstrates just how much insight can be gained from consulting with service-users to understand what does and does not work within a service provision. It is their lived experience, ideals, and perspectives that inform their market behaviours, so it is in the interest of service-providers to treat these service-users as the experts of market value. I propose that it is only these appraisers of services that can truly capture the difference between a service's benefits and its market value – whereby the *benefits* of a service are those which can be observed, felt, or measured to have changed within an individual's wellbeing, and *market value* describes the significance of this change when contextualised within its financial, temporal, and personal energy costs.

Where a Creative Health researcher or practitioner can be engulfed by their enthusiasm for a service's benefit and made blind to its chances of succeeding within a marketplace, a service-user is aware of the intricacies of their needs and the context which heightens or decreases the market value of this same service. Their insights offer an opportunity to improve the promotion of Creative Health services and reach people who are otherwise ostracised by the existing mental wellbeing system. In this context, market value is not all about financial benefit – rather it is important to the Creative Health movement because it captures the whole context of a service-user's choice to engage with an artistic provision or not.

By co-designing a Creative Health Communication Framework with members of the public, I was able to capture the way in which potential service-users understand and communicate about their own wellbeing stories. I designed around the promotional material which would feel most meaningful to them, in the hope that their search for support could one day be easier than my own. By placing *market relevancy* at the centre of this design, I have been able to offer readers a pragmatic solution to their promotional needs, rather than be led down an academic rabbit hole in search for supreme truthfulness.

Inherent in any activity related to improving precision in promotional communication, a natural biproduct is often improved precision in service design. Once service-users' needs are more clearly understood, the more a service-provider is able to respond and design around these needs – both practical and communicative. By treating service design as an iterative process, that this intricately linked to the planning, delivery, and evaluation of promotional communication, both researchers and service-providers in the field can seek to improve their market offering. This book is here to support them in that journey.

References

Baker, J.A., Canvin, K. and Berzins, K. (2019) The relationship between workforce characteristics and perception of quality of care in mental health: A qualitative study. *International Journal of Nursing Studies*, 100, p. 103412.

Davies, E. and Bucur, M. (2021) Consultation liaison to support efficient delivery of mental health care. *BJPsych Open*, 7(S1), pp. S317–S317.

GBD Mental Disorders Collaborators (2022) Global, regional, and national burden of 12 mental disorders in 204 countries and territories, 1990–2019: A systematic analysis for the Global Burden of Disease Study 2019. *The Lancet Psychiatry*, 9(2), pp. 137–150.

Kiely, B. et al. (2022) Effect of social prescribing link workers on health outcomes and costs for adults in primary care and community settings: A systematic review. *BMJ Open*, 12(10), p. e062951.

Kozera, K. (2022) *Yoga & Sound*. [Online] Surya Yoga Sound. Available from: https://www.instagram.com/p/Cg1WEi1s8E4/ [Accessed 01/10/2022].

Leicester Museum & Galleries (2022) *Health & Wellbeing – Leicester Museums*. Available from: https://www.leicestermuseums.org/learning-engagement/health-wellbeing/ [Accessed 19/11/2022].

NHS England and NHS Improvement (2020) *Managing Capacity and Demand Within Inpatient and Community Mental Health, Learning Disabilities and Autism Services for All Ages*. London: NHS England.

Palmer, W. et al. (2021) *Untapped? Understanding the Mental Health Clinical Support Workforce*. London: Nuffield Trust.

The Past Whispers. (2018) Directed by *Jane Hearst*. Hereford: Channel 4, Random Acts.

World Health Organisation (2021) *Depression*. [Online] World Health Organisation Fact Sheets. Available from: https://www.who.int/news-room/fact-sheets/detail/depression [Accessed 03/02/2022].

World Health Organization (2018) *Fact Sheet on Sustainable Development Goals (SDGs): Health Targets: Mental Health*. Copenhagen, Denmark: World Health Organization.

Chapter 2

Strategy, Sustainability, and the Context of Capitalism

One of the unique features of this book is that I conceptualise Creative Health as a key part of a wider healthcare system, as opposed to a fringe activity. Whilst the existence of Creative Health research and practice is not limited to formalised health systems, it's evolution, as a social movement, is largely shaped by the philosophies, cultures, and systematic limitations of these systems, necessitating our ability to understand them. Likewise, as the health needs of the general population evolve over time, so too do the systems that attempt to support them. Knowledge of these health needs informs the way that Creative Health researchers and practitioners prioritise their ambitions and communicate their strengths. By exploring the interplay between the philosophical biases and logistical pressures of healthcare systems, via an economic lens, this chapter aims to support Creative Health researchers and practitioners in improving their chances of gaining sustainable investment.

The Historical and Modern Context of the NHS

The NHS was conceptualised by the British economist William Henry Beveridge, who went on to play a central role in designing the welfare state in the UK. The Beveridge Report (1942) argued that the effects of the Industrial Revolution had been unevenly distributed. Namely, 'inadequate education, lack of social security, substandard housing and poor healthcare' (Hanlon and Carlisle, 2016, p. 20) were negatively affecting people's ability to contribute to the economy. It was proposed that with better health – the type offered through a nationalised healthcare service – people would become more active members in the economy. This shows that even at the root of our socialist healthcare system there are financial incentives for providing good health.

The NHS was proposed by Beveridge as a 'free' system that separated access away from funding. Underlying this notion was the philosophy of Universalism – a concept which claimed it was not only morally ideal but also economically and socially beneficial to have universally healthy citizens (Titmuss, 2006, pp. 40–41). As I consider the concept of Universalism in the modern day, where social disadvantages are the largest predictor of health

DOI: 10.4324/9781003423317-4

inequality, I am motivated to consider how this looks in practice. Allen and Allen (2016) advocate for 'Proportionate Universalism' whereby 'actions to improve the conditions in which people are born, grow, live, work, and age should be universal, but implemented with increasing intensity according to position on the social gradient' (p. 29). A WHO report describes this as 'levelling-up the social gradient in health' (Marmot, World Health Organization and UCL Institute of Health Equity, 2014) and this has shaped policies such as the levelling up agenda of the UK government.

Another useful philosophical term to consider in relation to the NHS is Utilitarianism, which is broadly defined as the greatest good for the greatest number of people. In a universalist system, the question of the greatest good is an interesting dilemma. Depending on interpretation, different stakeholders may deem either *length of life* or *quality of life* as the priority in this system. So far, in a system dominated by the biomedical model of health, length of life has been prioritised. Yet, according to research (e.g., Marmot et al., 2020) quality of life has a causal effect on length of life, whilst the opposite is not necessarily true. This is one of the reasons I invite you to question how much the financial market shapes the application of Utilitarianism. In a capitalist society, the 'greatest good' is often categorised as the greatest amount of profit for stockholders, rather than inherent moral value to society. This is called 'stockholder utility'.

As internal markets and privatisation increasingly shape the delivery of care within the NHS, it is concepts like stockholder utility that threaten to overtake Universalism as the principle that dominates the system. Therefore, Creative Health professionals may not be able to use the universalist values of the original NHS system when pitching their projects in the modern day. Rather, to achieve success, services must be able to pitch the economic benefits proposed by the original system, that is, how will the care that services provide affect the ability of service-users to contribute to the economy post-care.

Economic principles also have a part to play in what is funded through the NHS. Economics differentiates between 'economic goods' which are scarce, and 'free goods' which implies there is enough to go around for everybody who wants them. Coskeran (2019) notes that the NHS 'is free for users but for economists it is not a free good. Scarce resources are used in providing healthcare so it is an economic good' (p. 2).

In the case of scarce resources, funding providers, like the NHS, are presented with the dilemma of how to allocate resources between members of a society. The decision of how to allocate resources is shaped by the type of economy that funders provide from. In the UK, our healthcare system is split between market economies, which are consumer and producer led, and planned/command economies, which are government led (Coskeran, 2019, p. 5). Our NHS attempts to give its citizens equal access to healthcare, yet, since the introduction of internal markets, private suppliers increasingly dictate healthcare priorities based on profitability rather than health priority (Ruane, 2016a).

By recognising the complex power play between public and private aspects of the NHS, it becomes clearer as to why it is difficult to pitch for funding, as providers must demonstrate both how they contribute to national welfare and their competitive advantage over other health providers. In other words, they must demonstrate originality and innovation in their methods, whilst also considering whether it is scalable and cost effective. Add to this the difficulties that the NHS is currently undergoing with underfunding and the hostile nature of this market becomes even clearer.

The NHS is struggling to maintain its current provisions due to financial strain. Explicitly, it requires 'an average real terms increase of around 4% in funding each year to carry on producing services as before [...] [but is receiving] an average of just 1%' (Ruane, 2016b, 2016c). Accordingly, investment in new provisions can only be undertaken if they replace an existing service or reduce the burden on that service. This is called the 'opportunity cost,' which describes the services or products that cannot be invested in when funding is allocated to a particular provision. When pitching with opportunity cost in mind, providers must demonstrate how they outperform the next best option. Creative Health providers, in this case, are not pitching for funding from an endless reserve, rather they are competing with other health-promoting services for priority.

In 2012, the Department of Health noted that '30% of the population account for 70% of the [healthcare] spend' (Department of Health, 2012, p. 3). This is a statistic that I still hear spoken about within Integrated Care Boards today. It actively shapes their perspective on commissioning, with the health needs of this 30% being prioritised, in an effort to reduce demand and, therefore, make savings in the long term. This was also a key motivating factor when NHS England created their Core20PLUS5 priority population strategy – a comprehensive summary of demographics who experience inequality, either in access to healthcare (such as POC mothers during pregnancy) or in their health outcomes (including the 20% most deprived population in the UK, based on the Index of Multiple Deprivation). Creative Health practitioners that respond to strategic documents like this are more likely to be listened to and collaborated with, as they become instrumental stakeholders in managing health outcomes and budgets.

By reviewing the NHS's approach to mental health in recent history, it can be concluded that mental health is either not deemed to be a priority over other services – perhaps because the importance of physical health is more entrenched – or that they simply do not have the funding to invest in this evolving health concern. To illustrate, mental health services account for only 9% of NHS's total budget spend (Committee of Public Accounts, 2023).

Investigating the impact this had on our mental health services at the turn of the millennia, I found that 'waiting times of several months [were] known to be commonplace (Mental Health Foundation, 2006) and in extreme cases waits of up to two years [had] been recorded' (Wooster, 2008, p. 4).

Due to this, the Improving Access to Psychological Therapies (IAPT) programme was launched, in 2008, 'to improve the quality and accessibility of mental health services in England' (Baker, 2020, p. 15). Whilst this saw an improvement in time waited for initial consultation, the average waiting time between the first and second treatments raised considerably, causing some to label these as 'hidden waiting lists' (Triggle, 2019), strategically created to mask an uncontrollable problem. In some areas of the UK, up to 47% of people who received IAPT treatment have not experienced an improvement and up to 67% do not move on to 'recovery' (Baker, 2020, p. 20).

The scope to improve these services is limited both financially and by the number of people specialised to deliver this style of provision. One of the reasons why social prescribing has been introduced into the mental health picture is that it broadens the type of specialists that the NHS has access to. However, the operation of this system currently requires providers to be self-funded, with the role of the NHS being in referring patients towards these services. In this case, Creative Health providers who intend to offer their services to users for free may be required to pitch for funding from charities or private providers. Some NHS Trusts are more meaningfully funding and embedding community chosen assets into their mental health transformation plans. However, with limited budgets available, even here, we are forced to consider the legacy of these transformational programmes and how their reach can continue to be developed.

Shifting Needs in Healthcare

Hanlon and Carlisle (2016) believe there to be four distinct waves of healthcare in the UK since the early 19th century. They explain that 'each wave arose as a response to historically, geographically, and culturally defined needs' (p. 20). The first wave was focused on causes of diseases in the physical setting such as 'overcrowding, lack of clean water and sanitation, poor nutrition, and a dire built environment' (p. 19). The second wave benefitted from increased technology and scientific findings to advance the response to naturally occurring diseases. In the third wave, healthcare moved away from short-term disruptions of health to long-term ailments and, with this change in the health environment, a greater breadth of health specialists contributed to health debates (Beaglehole et al., 2004). This went on to shape the fourth wave, which became concerned with risky behaviours relating to 'diet, exercise, tobacco, alcohol, and consumption of illegal drugs' (Hanlon and Carlisle, 2016, p. 20). I believe that it is this history of healthcare that created fertile ground for creativity to be considered a key aspect of health in the modern day. As our society learnt about the multifaceted nature of health, we developed the sophistication of our healthcare infrastructure and broadened our expectations of what health needs can be addressed. However, just as our knowledge of health has shifted through time, so too have our population's health needs – necessitating a continued innovation-based approach to care.

One aspect of this changing need is linked to our aging population. Indeed, in just 200 years, humans around the world have doubled their life expectancy (Roser, Ortiz-Ospina and Ritchie, 2019) with citizens of the UK rating within the top percentile. Whilst life expectancy has been going up, the number of years lived in poor health is also increasing. For example, 'in 2018–20 a female in England could expect to live 83.1 years, of which 19.3 years (23 per cent) would have been spent in "not good" health' (quote from Raleigh, 2022; latest version of dataset from Population Health Monitoring Team (ONS), 2024). Banerjee (2016) claims that by 2050 we can expect there to be more people aged over 85 than there will be those aged under 16. Considering this, he reflects, 'the system was designed to deliver a particular set of outcomes [...] The outcomes are [now] different, because the biggest section of people who need that care are different' (Timestamp:9:19–9:34). This shifting of needs adds a new dimension to the pressures that the NHS now experiences, which is why it is important for Creative Health stakeholders to be aware of these needs. For example, 'fall-related fractures cost the health and social care system £4.4 billion per year' – that's £4.4 billion that cannot be spent elsewhere, unless provisions contribute to this health concern. Consequently, Creative Health advocates benefit from positioning themselves as problem-solvers and strategic collaborators, helping to manage the raising pressures of the NHS, rather than conceptualising their peers as adversaries who will not align to their ambitions. It is important for them to recognise that their ambitions are limited by the financial restraints of the system and the evolving portfolio of needs that draw upon these resources, rather than the individual people that are given the responsibility of managing these resources.

Fortunately, thanks to the evolving evidence-base for Creative Health, advocates are able to align themselves to the concerns of healthcare commissioners, whilst still promoting the uptake of creative provisions. For example, in the Nordic Countries, research has been undertaken, at population level, which suggests that arts engagement is one of the key factors affecting our ability to live longer lives, as well as higher quality lives (Gordon-Nesbitt, 2015). In dementia care, the arts are having a big impact. For example, movement and dance have been shown to help to reduce the risk of developing dementia in around 4,000 people per year, representing an annual saving of over £149 million (Boardman et al., 2023, p. 10). A study of visual arts across England and Wales calculated a social return on investment (SROI) of between £3.20 and £6.62 for every £1 spent on arts interventions for dementia care (Jones, Windle and Edwards, 2018). In connection to frailty and falls prevention in the elderly, there are also areas for creative impact. For example, music listening has been linked to decreased risk of falls in hospital patients of an older age (Chabot et al., 2019). Moreover, in a report on Aesop's Dance for Health programme, it was reported that falls can be reduced by 58% by mixing dance with physiotherapy (Aesop, 2020). Moreover, 'analyses of longitudinal cohort data have shown that cultural engagement is associated with a reduced risk of becoming frail and a slower progression of frailty over time' (data from Rogers and Fancourt, 2020; quote from Fancourt, Warran and Aughterson, 2020).

Another new pressure upon the healthcare system is that of mental health. The World Health Organisation (2021) explains that depression is a leading global cause of disability worldwide. The Department of Health (2011) in the UK has concluded that 'mental ill health is the single largest cause of disability in the UK, contributing up to 22.8% of the total burden, compared to 15.9% for cancer and 16.2% for cardiovascular disease'. Moreover, 'mental health problems in the under 65s account for almost half of NHS diagnosis' (APPG on Arts, Health and Wellbeing, 2017, p. 12). In research by Age UK, which assessed 15,000 UK residents aged 60 and above, 'creative and cultural participation was the single factor that contributed the most out of all 40 of the factors found to significantly contribute to wellbeing' (Archer et al., 2018, p. 3), suggesting a good fit for the Creative Health movement, when it comes to responding to mental health and wellbeing.

In a final contemplation about our current 'wave' of health, we can return to Hanlon and Carlisle (2016), who propose:

> Many of the health problems which cause the greatest concern today are [...] an emergent manifestation of our late modern culture rather than manifestations of diseases caused by known pathogens. [...] [They] reflect an 'inner world' – the realm of our individual consciousness, beliefs, and motivations – that is struggling to cope with modern life.
>
> (p. 20)

Evidence suggests there is much truth to Hanlon and Carlisle's assertions. For example, it has been suggested that less than 10% of an individual's health is now determined by their access to medical healthcare (McGovern, Miller and Hughes-Cromwick, 2014). Moreover, you are now more likely to die of loneliness than either smoking or obesity (Lim, Holt-Lunstad and Badcock, 2020). But if our health needs are no longer distinguished by their link to diseases or biological conditions, how should we conceptualise the scope of the NHS's role in providing care? This is where I witness a key tension between health commissioners and cultural practitioners. Both are aware of these evolving needs, but the system is slower to adapt and the financial resources are not able to grow at the same speed as these needs.

Strategizing Market Power

Wherever Creative Health providers intend to receive their investment from, they benefit from clearly articulating their value in market terms. Through the research conducted for this book, I identified a tendency for Creative Health projects to use vague language to describe their value to users. I argue that whilst describing their value as 'improving wellbeing' is not incorrect in the broad sense, it risks their service being lost within a marketplace full of competing initiatives. Kim and Mauborgne (2015) propose that this leaves services in 'red ocean' territory – that is, bloodied with competition. Their *Blue Ocean Strategy* proposes that service-providers can move into uncontested market space by differentiating their service values from those of others.

Similarly, Porter (1980, 1985) suggests that attaining competitive advantage requires providers to choose both the *type* of competitive advantage they wish to reach and the *scope* within which they seek to reach it. This leaves them with four different types of market strategy to choose from. These strategies are 1) Differentiation Leadership, 2) Cost Leadership, 3) Differentiation Focus, and 4) Cost Focus. Without this, companies become 'stuck in the middle' – a position void of strategic strength.

Cost Leadership describes the ability of a provider to outperform competitors on the price of equivalent products or services, within a dominant aspect of the market. Cost Focus, on the other hand, describes this same ability but within a more specialist segment of the market. For example, the NHS, as an organisation, offers cheaper medical care than any private provider, meaning that they hold a Cost Leadership in the UK. However, for people who want to skip waiting lists for services, such as neurodivergent diagnostic assessments or gender-affirming surgery for transgender people, then different private providers might compete on Cost Focus.

Differentiation Leadership and Differentiation Focus, on the other hand, describe the ability to outperform on quality or novelty. For example, mental health apps like Better Health compete with traditional face-to-face therapy services by making the counselling more accessible through digital sessions. Since their app is accessible to everyone, it competes on Differentiation Leadership. Services which target unique groups, such as culturally sensitive counselling providers for users that are LGBTQIA+ or POC, compete on Differentiation Focus. Differentiation services can be more expensive to access, but the added value is what distinguishes them within a market.

One of the reasons why the pharmaceutical side of the medical industry has proven to be strategically strong is due to its Cost Leadership. Its ability to produce highly replicable results means that a drug created to combat a disease in one sample of people can then be used by a multitude of other people to combat the same disease. By producing a highly replicable result, the ability to scale – that is, to produce more product whilst reducing the man-hours per unit of product – allows for pharmaceutical medicine, in theory, to be highly cost efficient. These services can be compared to the labour-intensive practices of the arts, which cannot be truly scaled, and questions can be presented in relation to the cost-to-benefit ratios of each offering.

As we begin to consider the preventative power of many Creative Health provisions, along with the potential for long-term effectiveness, there are now opportunities to begin challenging this perception. Alternatively, members of the Creative Health industry could choose to readdress the scalability of their provisions. One means of achieving this is by including technology within service design. To demonstrate the potential for technology in the health market, we can refer to Calm – 'the leading mental wellness and meditation app' (Ceci, 2021) – which 'generated more than 23 million U.S. dollars in IAP revenues worldwide' in the first quarter of 2021 (Ceci, 2021). Incorporating technology would likely lose some of the fluidity of creative activity and artistic thinking, so a key rationale for what service-users can benefit in this case would be recommended. However, this type of revenue, if drawn into a Creative Health business, could be used to fund additional in-person services that are free or affordable at the point of access.

Competing on Cost Leadership is not the only way for Creative Health providers to achieve strategic advantage. Considering the wide differences in philosophy and approach, explored earlier in this chapter, there may be other strategies that provide a stronger fit. The case set forwards by some Creative Health researchers is that by implementing arts provision in areas in which medicine is weak, the arts can produce cost savings. This segmenting of healthcare by specialism would produce a strategy of Cost Focus. Opportunities for Cost Focus include arts in hospitals and dementia care.

Due to the funding gap that the NHS is currently experiencing – between the cost of increasing demand and the money available to finance that care – it has been led towards a strategy of 'efficiency savings,' which involves, among other things, reducing the amount of time patients remain in hospital beds (Anandaciva, 2022). Evolving literature poses that visual art is capable of improving hospital patients' experience of pain and distress, as well as reducing their length of recovery (Lankston et al., 2010). Should this be true, then a case could be made for the role that art can play in helping hospitals to meet their efficiency quotas.

Moreover, in 2017, the APPG on Arts Health and Wellbeing noted that 'the annual cost of dementia to the UK is £23.3bn, which is more than the combined cost of treating cancer, heart disease and stroke' (APPG on Arts, Health and Wellbeing, 2017, p. 12). They argued that 'arts engagement can boost brain function and improve the recall of personal memories' (APPG on Arts, Health and Wellbeing, 2017, p. 12). This is supported by research elsewhere which has demonstrated the link between visual art therapy and cognitive function, with statistically significant results in the improvement of cognitive function after engagement (Masika, Yu and Li, 2020). Using arts in this way - to prevent the reliance of dementia patients on care homes and hospital treatment - as well as maintaining cognitive function of those receiving care to an extent that they do not require complex care, would arguably have a knock-on effect of reducing the costs associated with care. The arts also play a role in better researching and understanding experiences of dementia (Camic et al., 2021; Harding et al., 2021), so that more proficient care systems can be designed.

Analysing cost-related strategies further, it could be argued that since the existing health industry, in fact, depends on a large labour-heavy workforce, cost effectiveness is not the real indicator of its success. If we readdress the historical context for medicine's popularisation, then we see that it was not only subjected to a lens of financial efficiency but also wrapped in a narrative of science being effective, powerful, and ground-breaking. Through this lens, we may consider the medical industry not to be one of Cost Leadership, but rather Differentiation Leadership, as the breakthroughs of medicine offered control over health to unprecedented levels. Now, as we discover the limitations of medicine, we can reconsider the place of alternative provisions within these pockets of limitation. Here, there is plentiful opportunity for the arts to build a strategy of differentiation.

As I mentioned in the previous chapter, studies which emphasise the differentiation benefits of Creative Health practices, often focus on vulnerable groups, such as young people or the elderly. This would suggest that they are seeking a Differentiation Focus strategy based on the ability of the arts to support those with the highest social and mental health needs. This works fantastically well within a research space, where clear measurable demographics improve the chances of funding. However, within the private market, the strategy of Differentiation Focus is typically dependent on targeting a demographic with large buying power. Vulnerable groups do not typically have this power, meaning that providers become reliant on charities, the NHS, and community groups – all of which have limited grant money available.

In contrast, if providers were to use the information from the research evidenced in this chapter, they can demonstrate that there is a strong user demand for mental health services throughout the country. Importantly, this includes those coming from demographics typically associated with wealth. Whilst evidence certainly suggests that those at the bottom end of the socio-economic ladder struggle the most (Marmot et al., 2020), the Creative Health movement can use the resources afforded through wealthier clients to create a costing structure that draws money from those with large buying power, whilst still supporting those who are more vulnerable, thereby making it more sustainable. This would be a strategy of Differentiation Leadership.

Final Thoughts...

Throughout this chapter, I have demonstrated that the connection between inherent/moral value of Creative Health and the promotion of market value is a complex negotiation, particularly within the hostile environment of the UK's present healthcare market. Creative Health provisions exist outside of this system, whether it be via cultural commissioners or embedded within communities themselves as unlabelled, self-led practices. But, with an increase of Creative Health practitioners hoping to receive funding from the NHS, it is important to recognise that within different systems come different restrictions, philosophies, and strategic priorities. Now that some of those differences have been addressed, I will go on to explore the language-based tensions that shape the collaboration of health and cultural partners with members of the public.

References

Aesop (2020) *Dance to Health. Phase 1 Roll-out 'Test and Learn' Evaluation Report.* Oxfordshire: Aesop.

Allen, J. and Allen, M. (2016) The social determinants of health, empowerment, and participation. In: Clift, S. and Camic, P.M. (eds.) *Oxford Textbook of Creative Arts, Health, and Wellbeing: International Perspectives on Practice, Policy, and Research.* Oxford Textbooks in Public Health. Oxford, United Kingdom: Oxford University Press, pp. 27–34.

Anandaciva, S. (2022) *The Pritchard Challenge: The Next NHS Efficiency Drive.* [Online] The Kings Fund. Available from: https://www.kingsfund.org.uk/insight-and-analysis/blogs/pritchard-challenge-next-nhs-efficiency-drive [Accessed 26/10/2024].

APPG on Arts, Health and Wellbeing (2017) *Creative Health: The Arts for Health and Wellbeing.* London: All Party Parliamentary Group on Arts, Health and Wellbeing.

Archer, L. et al. (2018) *Creative and Cultural Activities and Wellbeing in Later Life.* Oxfordshire: Age UK.

Baker, C. (2020) *Mental Health Statistics for England: Prevalence, Services and Funding.* London: House of Commons.

Banerjee, J. (2016) *Living to Die.* [online] YouTube. Available at: https://www.youtube.com/watch?v=KDfqZWG4rUE [Accessed 02/12/2018].

Beaglehole, R. et al. (2004) Public health in the new era: Improving health through collective action. *The Lancet*, 363(9426), pp. 2084–2086.

Beveridge, W. (1942) *Social Insurance and Allied Services.* London: His Majesty's Stationery Office.

Boardman, R. et al. (2023) *Social Value of Movement and Dance.* London: Sport + Recreation Alliance.

Camic, P.M. et al. (2021) Developing poetry as a research methodology to further understand rarer forms of dementia. In: *Culture, Health and Wellbeing International Conference (CHW21) Research Proceedings. Culture, Health and Wellbeing International Conference (CHW21).* UK: Arts and Health South West.

Ceci, L. (2021) *Calm: Mobile App Global IAP Revenues 2021.* [Online] Statista. Available from: https://www.statista.com/statistics/1243071/calm-iap-revenues-worldwide/ [Accessed 20/01/2022].

Chabot, J. et al. (2019) Decreased Risk of Falls in Patients Attending Music Sessions on an Acute Geriatric Ward: Results from a Retrospective Cohort Study. *BMC Complementary and Alternative Medicine*, 19(1), p. 76.

Committee of Public Accounts (2023) *Progress in Improving NHS Mental Health Services*. [Online] UK Parliament. Available from: https://publications.parliament.uk/pa/cm5803/cmselect/cmpubacc/1000/report.html [Accessed 29/02/2024].

Coskeran, T. (2019) *Economics: A Complete Introduction*. Revised and updated edition. London: Teach Yourself.

Department of Health (2011) *No Health Without Mental Health: A Cross-Government Mental Health Outcomes Strategy for People of All Ages. Supporting Document – The Economic Case for Improving Efficiency and Quality in Mental Health*. London: HM Government.

Department of Health (2012) *Long Term Conditions Compendium of Information: Third Edition*. London: Department of Health – Long-term conditions.

Fancourt, D., Warran, K. and Aughterson, H. (2020) *Evidence Summary for Policy: The Role of Arts in Improving Health & Wellbeing*. London: UCL.

Gordon-Nesbitt, R. (2015) *Exploring the Longitudinal Relationship Between Arts Engagement and Health*. Manchester: Arts For Health.

Hanlon, P. and Carlisle, S. (2016) The fifth wave of public health and the contributions of culture and the arts. In: Clift, S. and Camic, P.M. (eds.) *Oxford Textbook of Creative Arts, Health, and Wellbeing: International Perspectives on Practice, Policy, and Research*. Oxford Textbooks in Public Health. Oxford, United Kingdom: Oxford University Press, pp. 19–26.

Harding, E. et al. (2021) Developing a drawing-based method to capture and communicate experiences of rare dementias. In: *Culture, Health and Wellbeing International Conference (CHW21) Research Proceedings. Culture, Health and Wellbeing International Conference (CHW21)*. UK: Arts and Health South West.

Jones, C., Windle, G. and Edwards, R.T. (2018) Dementia and imagination: A social return on investment analysis framework for art activities for people living with dementia. *The Gerontologist*, [Online] Available from: https://doi.org/10.1093/geront/gny147 [Accessed 13/12/2023].

Kim, W.C. and Mauborgne, R. (2015) *Blue Ocean Strategy: How to Create Uncontested Market Space and Make the Competition Irrelevant*. Expanded edition. Boston, Massachusetts: Harvard Business Review Press.

Lankston, L. et al. (2010) Visual Art in Hospitals: Case Studies and Review of the Evidence. *Journal of the Royal Society of Medicine*, 103(12), pp. 490–499.

Lim, M.H., Holt-Lunstad, J. and Badcock, J.C. (2020) Loneliness: Contemporary Insights into Causes, Correlates, and Consequences. *Social Psychiatry and Psychiatric Epidemiology*, 55(7), pp. 789–791.

Marmot, M., World Health Organization and UCL Institute of Health Equity (eds.) (2014) *Review of Social Determinants and the Health Divide in the WHO European Region: Final Report*. Copenhagen: World Health Organization, Regional Office for Europe.

Marmot, M. et al. (2020) *Health Equity in England: The Marmot Review 10 Years On*. London: Institute of Health Equity.

Masika, G.M., Yu, D.S.F. and Li, P.W.C. (2020) Visual art therapy as a treatment option for cognitive decline among older adults. A systematic review and meta-analysis. *Journal of Advanced Nursing*, 76(8), p. jan.14362.

McGovern, L., Miller, G. and Hughes-Cromwick, P. (2014) *The Relative Contribution of Multiple Determinants to Health*. Michigan: Project HOPE.

Mental Health Foundation (2006) *We Need to Talk: The Case for Psychological Therapies on the NHS. London: MHF*. London: Mental Health Foundation.

Population Health Monitoring Team (ONS) (2024). Health state life expectancy, all ages, UK. [online] Office for National Statistics. Available at: https://www.ons.gov.uk/peoplepopulationandcommunity/healthandsocialcare/healthandlifeexpectancies/datasets/healthstatelifeexpectancyallagesuk [Accessed 6/01/2025].

Porter, M.E. (1980) *Competitive Strategy: Techniques for Analyzing Industries and Competitors*. New York: Free Press.

Porter, M.E. (1985) *Competitive Advantage: Creating and Sustaining Superior Performance*. New York: London: Free Press; Collier Macmillan.

Raleigh, V. (2022) *What is Happening to Life Expectancy in England?*. [Online] The Kings Fund. Available from: https://www.kingsfund.org.uk/insight-and-analysis/long-reads/whats-happening-life-expectancy-england#:~:text=Compared%20with%202019%2C%20life%20expectancy,in%20the%20past%20two%20decades [Accessed 09/02/2024].

Rogers, N.T. and Fancourt, D. (2020) Cultural engagement is a risk-reducing factor for frailty incidence and progression Neupert, S. (ed.). *The Journals of Gerontology: Series B*, 75(3), pp. 571–576.

Roser, M., Ortiz-Ospina, E. and Ritchie, H. (2019) *Life Expectancy*. Available from: https://ourworldindata.org/life-expectancy [Accessed 11/11/2020].

Ruane, S. (2016a) Market reforms and privatisation in the English National Health Service/Mercado reforma y privatizacion en el Sistema Nacional de Salud ingles. *Cuadernos de Relaciones Laborales*, (2), p. 263+.

Ruane, S. (2016b) TEDx Talk Leicester Salon: Health of the Nation: Should we care? [TEDx]. https://campaignagainstnhsprivatization.files.wordpress.com/2011/11/tedxtalk-should-we-care.pdf [Accessed 16/05/2022].

Ruane, S. (2016c) *NHS - On the Wrong Path*. [online] YouTube. Available at: https://www.youtube.com/watch?v=saeTTzlsfh0 [Accessed 16/05/2022].

Titmuss, R. (2006) Universalism versus selection. In: Pierson, C. and Castles, F.G. (eds.) *The Welfare State Reader*. Cambridge: Polity, pp. 40–49.

Triggle, N. (2019) Hidden waits 'leave mental health patients in limbo'. *BBC News*, 5 December. https://www.bbc.co.uk/news/health-50658007

Wooster, E. (2008) *While We Are Waiting*. London: Mental Health Foundation.

World Health Organisation (2021) *Depression*. [Online] World Health Organisation Fact Sheets. Available from: https://www.who.int/news-room/fact-sheets/detail/depression [Accessed 03/02/2022].

Chapter 3

Modern-Day Healthcare and Conceptualisations of Mental Health

In the introduction to this book, I explained that I make a distinction between 'mental health,' which is a term used frequently within clinical settings, and 'mental wellbeing,' which is denoted as something more holistic and personalised, but not always within the remit of healthcare. In this chapter, I explore some of the reasons why this distinction is upheld by medical professionals and why it may need to be challenged as our healthcare system develops and the expectations of the public shift. To quote City Lit, Leicester, this might be a movement towards discussions of 'Mental Wealth' and the place that creativity can have in supporting it.

Positivist and Humanistic Conceptualisation of Mental Health

To begin, let us investigate common descriptors of mental health within healthcare and assess how these politically charged labels impact the delivery of care.

The NHS collects 34 common mental illnesses on its website, including bipolar disorder, clinical depression, post-traumatic stress disorder, and schizophrenia (NHS, 2021). These unified categorisations give medical professionals a sense of scope regarding symptoms; symptoms which they attempt to treat using biological evidence and related medicine. For example, the *monoamine hypothesis* considers serotonin deficiency to be the cause of depression. Accordingly, Selective Serotonin Reuptake Inhibitors (SSRI's) – the most common type of anti-depressant used in UK – are built to increase serotonin activity. These medications do not treat the underlying causes of serotonin deficiency – which may be natural bodily responses to external pressures in the social world – they simply manage the symptom experienced as a result of these pressures.

There is research into the success of mental illness medications – particularly papers which have not been funded by pharmaceutical organisations – which clearly shows that the long-term mental health of individuals on medication is poorer than those with limited or no use of it (e.g., Hengartner et al., 2019).

DOI: 10.4324/9781003423317-5

This has led health professionals to challenge the way that mental health and wellbeing are conceptualised and responded to within the UK healthcare system. Warren (2020), for example, argues that 'widespread prescribing has not reduced mental disability or suicide [...] [so] given limited efficacy and long-term safety concerns, the current level of UK prescribing is a major public health concern' (m3200). What is particularly important, from a market viewpoint, is that the NHS incurs major costs due to the prescription of unnecessary medicines such as these (Davies et al., 2022), creating a gap in the market for more cost-effective solutions that approach mental health and wellbeing from a different perspective.

Provisions which use more holistic definitions of wellbeing – including a significant proportion of Creative Health services – move away from the treatment of chemical imbalances towards goals such as the resolution of things such as power imbalances (Kinderman, 2021). This reprioritising of aspects of mental health and wellbeing, away from the psychoanalytical side of mental illness towards an account that is more than the absence of symptoms, can be understood as a shift towards humanistic psychology (Fancourt, 2017, p. 31). Schneider, Pierson and Bugental (2014) label humanistic psychology as a holistic approach to mentality; 'a rich mosaic consisting of each of the emerging trends but threaded throughout by the depth, breadth, and pathos of intimate human experience' (p. xvii). What I believe to be critical within this definition is that humanistic psychology does not reject the importance of psychoanalytical input, it simply places importance on contextualising this input alongside other unique findings from different disciplinary perspectives. For this reason, House, Kalisch and Maidman (2017) argue that humanistic values 'remain the strongest bulwark that we have against the triumph of technocratic scientism, soulless materialism, and the march of the inhuman' (p. 8), a sentiment that many emerging Creative Health practitioners appear to carry an affinity with.

Humanistic psychology was recognised as a distinct field in 1961 when Maslow and Sutich launched *The Journal of Humanistic Psychology*. Maslow is renowned for creating a hierarchy of needs. Whilst these needs are often depicted in terms of a pyramid, Bridgman, Cummings and Ballard (2019) show that it was not Maslow who situated these needs within a pyramid, and Kaufman (2022) argues that this pyramid has distorted our understanding of how integrative humanistic approaches are intended to be applied.

Kaufman warns that wellbeing should not be treated like a video game, whereby individuals can level up and win (pp. xxiii–3), and Rowan (1999) suggests that hierarchies of need are better understood via the metaphor of a Russian doll (p. 130), whereby each level of need is encapsulated within another. Here, 'higher' needs can transcend basic needs once they have been mastered within specific contexts, but as individuals move between environments, alter their values, or encounter new challenges they are wise to return to 'lower needs' until they have reorientated (Rowan, 1999, p. 130). Kaufman (2022) suggests that an implication of Maslow's theory is that an individual who attempts to grow too quickly will lack the ability to meet their full growth potential. For example, he insists that 'doing the downward-facing dog yoga pose every morning won't magically give you a deep sense of self-worth and connection with others' (xxxi) and that we should instead 'draw strength from our hardships, and work toward greater integration of our whole being' (xxxii). Likewise, I argue that many Creative Health provisions, which are deemed to support wellbeing, are not catch-all solutions to feeling happy and well at all times, rather they contribute to the fullness of being human and our never-ending pursuit of self-knowledge. This is important to distinguish against the biomedical approach to mental health, whereby medicine can sometimes be treated as the first and final response.

These considerations of humanistic psychology demonstrate, firstly, that both biological and physiological needs are important aspects of the human experience but are far from descriptive of the whole wellbeing picture. Secondly, they challenge the notions of psychoanalytic theory, which believes there is a single 'best' way of being and that this is a state that can be reached and sustained. Accordingly, in this book, I take an approach to wellbeing which incorporates different aspects of fulfilment and I do not treat service-users' journeys as a linear up-hill climb towards happiness. I acknowledge that moments of hardship are often integral parts of a long-term wellbeing story and, therefore, challenges should not be entirely avoided but, instead, better supported to maximise learning, development, and long-term eudaimonia. In this context, I use 'eudaimonia' to refer to the act of being content and the pursuit of long-term fulfilment over short-term pleasures.

Rowan (1999) describes the discrepancies between conceptualisations of mental health and wellbeing as a negotiation between *abundance motivation* and *deficiency motivation*. This rationale is mirrored within modern-day debates on the differences between surviving and thriving where 'to survive means to continue to live or exist in spite of danger, whereas to thrive means to grow, develop and prosper' (Walsh, 2017). The COVID-19 pandemic shaped the awareness of wellbeing held by citizens of the UK, whereby this debate between surviving and thriving was at the centre of wellbeing considerations. This demonstrates that the humanistic model of psychology is particularly relevant to the current political climate, further validating my use of it within this book.

Despite the timeliness of humanistic psychology, there is, however, an ongoing debate about which approach to care is more appropriate. For some, the parameters of stress are important, as some types of stress can be beneficial for wellbeing. Specifically, there is a difference between eustress which is positive and distress which is negative. Since Maslow's hierarchy of needs has been distorted within its popular pyramid depiction, advocates of positivist psychology – whereby empirical methods of observation and verification make stricter judgements about what is true or serviceable within the field of wellbeing – challenge humanistic psychology's ability to account for these distinctions.

Adding to this, medical providers that are traditionally minded prefer the measurability of biological indicators as these parameters provide them with a clear indication of their role. I argue that whilst this makes their role manageable, we should challenge the presumption that biological functions are responsible for the majority of mental health issues. This is supported by other humanistic advocates. Filer (2019), for example, questions whether extreme acts associated with mental ill-health conditions (such as schizophrenia) are actually very normal responses to extreme pressures and are, therefore, more commonly the result of social inequalities. Considering mental health and wellbeing at large, I agree that a large proportion of people who are experiencing mental health difficulties, experience such through social factors that they face. Whether this be increasing financial pressures, the attempt to keep up with the intensification of interaction caused by technology, mounting political and economic disasters, environmental destruction and decreased access to nature, increased isolation, pervasive consumerisation, or other factors. This brings me onto my next topic of discussion: health inequality and the social determinants of health.

Health Inequality and the Social Determinants of Health

In 2010, a national report, referred to as The Marmot Review, was released detailing the social determinants of health found in the UK (Marmot et al., 2010). This report evidenced that social conditions were one of the most deterministic influencers of health in the UK, affecting total years lived, number of disability-free years lived, and degree of overall wellbeing (Marmot et al., 2010). 'In England, those who live in the most deprived areas spend 17 years longer with a disabling illness than those who live in the richest areas, and they live on average seven years less' (Allen and Allen, 2016, p. 27).

In 2020, a follow-up report was released (Marmot, Allen, Boyce, et al., 2020) which confirmed these findings and highlighted the lack of progress made in British society over the 10-year interval. I consider these research findings on social inequality and its impact on mental health and wellbeing to be of interest to my research, as it points towards which pockets of the public are being most unheard or underrepresented within the current wellbeing 'market' – that is, clinical mental health programmes.

In considering health inequality, a distinction must be made between absolute and relative poverty. Wilkinson and Pickett (2010) propose 'almost everything – from life expectancy to mental illness, violence to illiteracy – is affected not by how wealthy a society is, but how equal it is' (p. cover). This theory was tested during the pandemic, with regional inequalities and infection rates suggesting there is great truth to this claim (Tubadji, Webber and Boy, 2020). Researchers warn that the pandemic not only highlighted inequality, but significantly heightened it (e.g., Pierce et al., 2020), posing extra concern for future health services. Indeed, Patel, et al. (2020) explain that UK policymakers disregarded the vulnerability of those who were most economically disadvantaged throughout the pandemic. This led many to challenge the government's plan to 'build back better' (Sunak, 2021), which had an economic focus, calling instead that we 'build back fairer' (e.g., Marmot, Allen, Goldblatt, et al., 2020; D'Ambruoso, Abbott and Binagwaho, 2021).

From this, it is clear how much the context of lifestyle and societal value systems have a part to play, not only in how we experience mental wellbeing but also in how we market it. Increasingly, professionals in the field of wellbeing are challenging the assumption that individuals should be held entirely responsible for their wellbeing, recognising, instead, the role that governments, policymakers, economic systems, and healthcare practices have to play (The Centre for Social Determinants of Health, 2008; Donkin et al., 2018).

Whilst academic knowledge on inequalities and mental wellbeing has existed for quite some time, it was the media coverage of the topic during the COVID-19 pandemic (e.g., Goldin, 2021) that finally drew this knowledge towards the forefront of public awareness. This engagement of the public shapes the way that the market responds to these issues, increasing the chances of social provisions reaching their target users.

Public and Holistic Conceptualisations of Wellbeing

In addition to the heightened awareness of inequality, recent years have also witnessed growing public interest in mental wellbeing thanks to shifts in social attitudes. One way that this can be measured is through the use of the hashtag #MentalHealth on social media platforms. On X (formerly twitter), for example, the hashtag #MentalHealth is used over 270 times per hour, with a hashtag exposure of almost 2 million viewers (RiteTag, 2020).

With the increase in online communication about mental health, the lines between everyday mental wellbeing and mental health diagnosis have – at least in the public's perception – become blurred. In fact, nearly half of adults think that they have had a diagnosable mental health condition at some point in their life (NHS Digital, 2016). This shows that it is not only the medical industry that is shifting its conceptualisation of mental health but also the members of the public that it serves. This recognition is important as this book prioritises engagement with service-users over consultation with medical professionals, and it is vital that the philosophical backdrop of my research is facilitative of their viewpoints and needs.

One powerful organisation which is advancing this shift towards a comprehensive definition of mental health and wellbeing is the World Health Organization (WHO). Constituted in 1948, WHO has a primary function 'to direct and coordinate international health within the United Nations system' (World Health Organisation, 2020, para. 8). Their impact is felt throughout the globe due to their incredible size; 'working with 194 Member States, across six regions, and from more than 150 offices' (para. 4). Their support shows that despite a traditional imbalance of power towards psychoanalytical approaches in the market, there are powerful stakeholders pushing towards a humanistic agenda. Significantly, WHO understands wellbeing to be situational, political, relating to culture and economy (World Health Organisation, 2020). In the Ottawa Charter of 1986, they maintained that health is 'a resource for everyday life, not the object of living [...] a positive concept emphasizing social and personal resources, as well as physical capacities' (World Health Organisation, 1986).

This definition of health can be described as the biopsychosocial model, meaning that it describes 'a state of complete physical, mental and social well-being and not merely an absence of disease or infirmity' (World Health Organisation, 1946). In comparison, a focus on biological indicators can be described as the biomedical model of health.

Fancourt (2017) explains that the biomedical model used to encompass our approach to healthcare (p. 23). Our shift from this model was due to evidence arising from public health on the impact of social causes of disease, psychoanalytic theories that related the mind to physical illness, and research from behavioural medicine on the relationship between behavioural risk factors and health (Fancourt, 2017, p. 28). These models were officially combined by George Engel in 1977. He described the biopsychosocial model as 'a blueprint for research, a framework for teaching, and a design for action in the real world of healthcare' (Engel, 1977, p. 1). Brown explains, however, that the biopsychosocial model was not entirely new; with every large advancement – such as Pasteur's Germ Theory – public consciousness is simply directed to a specific innovation to the point where it 'overwhelmed the rest of the field' (Ader and Brown, 2004).

Having investigated the negative effects that siloed responses can have on the shape of modern medical care, I suggest that the prevailing dominance of the biomedical model should be considered unjust. With increased literature and technology supporting the biopsychosocial model, I argue it is within our best interests to sustain an equilibrium in health modelling in the future – specifically, one that gives equal weight to medicine, community work, and Creative Health practices. The importance of this chapter is to demonstrate how power can fluctuate in who gets to define mental health and wellbeing, and how the limitations of one viewpoint place limitations on the sophistication of our care responses. It is my hope that this book can contribute towards the maintenance of the biopsychosocial view of mental health and wellbeing, using its Creative Health Communication Framework, and that this balance of opinion will improve the resonance of the services we can provide across the UK and internationally.

References

Ader, R. and Brown, T. (2004) *The Biopsychosocial Model: Interdisciplinarity in Science and Medicine*. [Interview – online] University of Rochester. Available at: https://sa.rochester.edu/jur/issues/fall2004/interview-ader_brown.pdf [Accessed 25/11/2020].

Allen, J. and Allen, M. (2016) The social determinants of health, empowerment, and participation. In: Clift, S. and Camic, P.M. (eds.) *Oxford Textbook of Creative Arts, Health, and Wellbeing: International Perspectives on Practice, Policy, and Research*. Oxford Textbooks in Public Health. Oxford, United Kingdom: Oxford University Press, pp. 27–34.

Bridgman, T., Cummings, S. and Ballard, J. (2019) Who built Maslow's pyramid? A history of the creation of management studies' most famous symbol and its implications for management education. *Academy of Management Learning & Education*, 18(1), pp. 81–98.

D'Ambruoso, L., Abbott, P. and Binagwaho, A. (2021) Building back fairer in public health policy requires collective action with and for the most vulnerable in society. *BMJ Global Health*, 6(3), p. e005555.

Davies, J. et al. (2022) The costs incurred by the NHS in England due to the unnecessary prescribing of dependency-forming medications. *Addictive Behaviors*, 125, p. 107143.

Donkin, A. et al. (2018) Global action on the social determinants of health. *BMJ Global Health*, 3(Suppl 1), p. e000603.

Engel, G. (1977) The need for a new medical model: A challenge for biomedicine. *Science*, 196(4286), pp. 129–136.

Fancourt, D. (2017) *Arts in Health: Designing and Researching Interventions*. First edition. Oxford; New York, NY: Oxford University Press.

Filer, N. (2019) *This Book Will Change Your Mind About Mental Health: A Journey into the Heartland of Psychiatry*. London: Faber & Faber.

Goldin, I. (2021) Covid-19 has made fighting inequality more critical than ever. *The Financial Times*, 6 September.

Hengartner, M.P. et al. (2019) Antidepressant Use During Acute Inpatient Care Is Associated With an Increased Risk of Psychiatric Rehospitalisation Over a 12-Month Follow-Up After Discharge. *Frontiers in Psychiatry*, 10, p. 79.

House, R., Kalisch, D. and Maidman, J. (eds.) (2017) *Humanistic Psychology: Current Trends and Future Prospects*. First edition. London; New York: Routledge.

Kaufman, S.B. (2022) *Transcend: The New Science of Self-Actualization*. London: Sheldon Press.

Kinderman, P. (2021) From chemical imbalance to power imbalance: A macropsychology perspective on mental health. In: MacLachlan, M. and McVeigh, J. (eds.) *Macropsychology*. Cham: Springer International Publishing, pp. 29–44.

Marmot, M., Allen, J., Boyce, T., et al. (2020) *Health Equity in England: The Marmot Review 10 Years On*. London: Institute of Health Equity. https://www.instituteofhealthequity.org/resources-reports/marmot-review-10-years-on/the-marmot-review-10-years-on-full-report.pdf

Marmot, M., Allen, J., Goldblatt, P., et al. (2020) *Build Back Fairer: The COVID-19 Marmot Review. The Pandemic, Socioeconomic and Health Inequalities in England*. London: Institute of Health Equity. https://www.health.org.uk/reports-and-analysis/reports/build-back-fairer-the-covid-19-marmot-review

Marmot, M. et al. (2010) *Fair Society, Healthy Lives: The Marmot Review*. London: Institute of Health Equity. Available from: https://www.instituteofhealthequity.org/resources-reports/fair-society-healthy-lives-the-marmot-review/fair-society-healthy-lives-full-report-pdf.pdf [Accessed 26/10/2020].

NHS (2021) *Mental Health Conditions*. Available from: https://www.nhs.uk/mental-health/conditions/ [Accessed 30/09/2022].

NHS Digital (2016) *Adult Psychiatric Morbidity Survey: Survey of Mental Health and Wellbeing, England, 2014*. London: NHS.

Patel, J.A. et al. (2020) Poverty, inequality and COVID-19: The forgotten vulnerable. *Public Health*, 183, pp. 110–111.

Pierce, M. et al. (2020) Mental health before and during the COVID-19 pandemic: A longitudinal probability sample survey of the UK population. *The Lancet Psychiatry*, 7(10), pp. 883–892.

RiteTag (2020) *Popular Hashtags for Mentalhealth on Twitter and Instagram*. Available from: https://ritetag.com/best-hashtags-for/mental%20health [Accessed 16/04/2020].

Rowan, J. (1999) Ascent and Descent in Maslow's Theory. *Journal of Humanistic Psychology*, 39(3), pp. 125–133.

Schneider, K.J., Pierson, J.F. and Bugental, J.F.T. (eds.) (2014) *The Handbook of Humanistic Psychology: Theory, Research, and Practice*. Second edition. Los Angeles: SAGE Publications, Inc.

Sunak, R. (2021) *Build Back Better: Our Plan for Growth*. London: HM Treasury.

The Centre for Social Determinants of Health (2008) *Closing the Gap in a Generation: Health Equity through Action on the Social Determinants of Health. Final Report of the Commission on Social Determinants of Health*. Geneva: World Health Organisation.

Tubadji, A., Webber, D.J. and Boy, F. (2020) Cultural and economic discrimination by the Great Leveller: The COVID-19 pandemic in the UK. *Centre for Economic Policy Research Press*, 13, pp. 48–67.

Walsh, M. (2017) *Surviving or Thriving*. [Online] Talk in the Bay Therapeutic Consultants. Available from: http://talkinthebay.co.uk/surviving-or-thriving/ [Accessed 17/05/2022].

Warren, J.B. (2020) The trouble with antidepressants: why the evidence overplays benefits and underplays risks—an essay by John B Warren. *BMJ*, 370, p. m3200.

Wilkinson, R.G. and Pickett, K. (2010) *The Spirit Level: Why Equality Is Better for Everyone; [With a New Chapter Responding to Their Critics]*. Publ. with a new postscript. London: Penguin Books.

World Health Organisation (1946) *Preamble to the Constitution of WHO as adopted by the International Health Conference*.

World Health Organisation (1986) *The Ottawa Charter for Health Promotion*. Ottawa: The World Health Organisation.

World Health Organisation (2020) *Who We Are: Constitution*. Available from: https://www.who.int/about/who-we-are/constitution [Accessed 24/10/2020].

Chapter 4

Categorisation and Power within the Field of Creative Health

The Creative Health agenda is shaped by a social movement, an evolving field of research, and a growth of activity across multiple, overlapping industries, all of which are committed to advocating for the benefits of creativity. At the time of writing this book, the field is in an exciting period of development, as more and more evidence is being gathered on the benefits of Creative Health interventions. Thanks to this mounting evidence, great progress has been made politically, practically, and in policy development.

In the UK, the field has garnered political support, such as the All-Party Parliamentary Group (APPG) on Creative Health (previously the APPG on Arts, Health and Wellbeing). This has led to the creation of the National Centre for Creative Health (NCCH), as well as a number of Creative Health research centres, such as the World Health Organisation's (WHO) Collaborating Centre for Arts & Health, at University College London (UCL). Creative Health strategies, such as Birmingham City Council's Creative Public Health programme, are now being developed in teams across the UK. There is a strong and growing National Arts in Hospitals Network (NAHN). Moreover, there has been an introduction of strategic posts within the UK's National Healthcare System (NHS) spotlighting Creative Health and its place within collaborative care. These posts include the Social Prescribing and Creative Health Commissioning Development Manager in Gloucestershire ICB, the Arts & Health Programme Manager in West Yorkshire ICB, and the Strategic Lead for Live Well and Creative Health in Greater Manchester ICS.

Whilst this progress is thoroughly worthy of celebration, we need to be mindful of the consequences that follow from the field becoming more professionalised, such as the successes of the movement being scrutinised by a wider audience of stakeholders. It is for these reasons that I talk about Creative Health in terms of markets, services, goals, and industries – not to discredit the organic growth of grassroots activity, but to acknowledge the power relations that exist across the movement and to signal that the delivery of this activity is worthy of appropriate compensation/commissioning. In doing so, I pay recognition to the differences that arise between practitioner ideals and market restraints.

DOI: 10.4324/9781003423317-6

With that in mind, this chapter will look at some of the common categorisations used to describe Creative Health throughout the professionalised side of the movement. The frequency that this language is used throughout networking events and academic literature suggests an invisible power dynamic – one which prioritises these categorisations above others. My intension, throughout this chapter, is to begin to pick apart what those power relations might be. The topics I discuss are intended to provide an introductory exploration of power dynamics. This is not the whole picture of power in the movement – that depth of exploration would require a book in its own right – but it is enough to show that Creative Health is not born from equality. Furthermore, what this movement becomes in the future will be shaped by who we choose to be heard and how their voices are allowed to impact the design and delivery of provisions.

Creative Arts Therapies (CATs)

To better understand Creative Health labels and their significance, I begin with a comparison of formal and informal Creative Arts Therapies (CATs). Informed by counselling traditions, CATs seek to provide a creative counterpart to traditional therapy; one which is of equivalent repute. The leading practices within this movement are Art Therapy, Dramatherapy, and Music Therapy.

Art Therapy places emphasis on visual interpretations of the world and the different types of symbology that are implicit. Dramatherapy (including Puppetry) focuses on the roles that people play throughout their lived experience and how they relate or interact with others around them. Meanwhile, Music Therapy engages the brain's relational networks to simulate journeys and their emotional responses.

As pioneering arts forms within CAT, these practices carry the longest track record of quality research outputs and have formal qualifications associated with their practice. This has afforded them heightened respect within the field of Creative Health. Moreover, they are each regulated by external bodies. Specifically, 'anyone who refers to themselves as an Art Therapist, Dramatherapist or Music Therapist must be registered with the Health and Care Professions Council (HCPC)' (Mind, 2021, p. 5). This offers assurance to service-users that these practitioners are reaching a recognised standard of care and are using methods that are backed by evidence.

Body Work and Movement Therapies, such as Dance, are not yet registered forms of therapy but they are quickly working towards gaining comparable recognition and respect to the more established provisions. Movement Therapies explore embodiment and interrelated connection, and practitioners work with their service-users to heighten their literacy of non-verbal symbology. Whilst Dance Therapy is an unregistered type of therapy, professionals working in this specialism are encouraged to belong to professional bodies such as the Association for Dance Movement Psychotherapy UK (ADMP UK). This connection to a professional organisation affords them strength within the market when compared to other unregistered forms of therapy.

CATs are a particularly good indicator of market powers and interests, as inherent within their models is the belief that a practitioner can be trained into the correct way of using the arts for therapeutic purposes. It naturally follows that this formalisation of artistic practice assumes that artistic professionals trained within specific therapeutic models have more to offer a service-user than other artistic providers (see: Dileo and Bradt, 2009). Consequently, Parkinson (2018) explains that numerous arts professionals have reported that the validity of their work has been questioned by the public based on the inclusion or exclusion of the word therapist within their title.

These findings suggest that whilst scientifically led services are not the only recipients of power within the marketplace, they are a significant authority and they have shaped the perceptions of market users in relation to what constitutes as quality care. It is for this reason that many Creative Health advocates seek to challenge scientific hierarchies and politicised evaluation practices which restrict the ability of the arts to thrive.

Other CATs, such as Film Therapy, are still developing their standard practices, so are less respected by the scientific community (Cohen, Johnson and Orr, 2015). However, despite their market positioning, each of these mediums has been shown to carry unique wellbeing support features. For example, where Sculpture Therapy is built around the emotional resonance that is associated with tactile touch, Poetry Therapy builds upon metaphor and non-literal expressions of knowing. Other interesting examples include Textile Therapies, which are used to slow down the pace of movement in an individual's lifestyle and encourage sensory comfort, and Cinema-/Bibliotherapy, where a counsellor guides their client to watch a certain film or read a specific book so that, together, they can discuss the client's emotional response to the content. These are distinct from therapies such as Sandplay, where the focus is on the externalisation and disassembly of negative emotions, or Filmmaking Therapy, whereby individuals create filmic re-imaginings of their stories, negotiate meaning with a production cast/crew, and control trauma responses through the editing process.

What is particularly interesting about this is that many of these self-labelled 'therapies' do not lack ideas about what the strengths of their mediums are and how this can help with mental wellbeing, but they have chosen specifically to be more flexible and conceptual in their approach. Since the framework of modern-day therapies are more restrictive and precise than many of these practitioners intend for their own practice, their choice to self-label in terms of therapy might point towards an unconscious acknowledgement of the power that this language affords within a market or an active disagreement against limiting the term in this way.

Considering therapies more broadly, these practices can either utilise a pure arts approach or opt for a hybrid method. In the latter scenario, talking therapies and creative exploration are used alongside one another. Madden and Bloom (2004) distinguish between these two types of artistic delivery by asserting that 'art as therapy' is an approach which puts weight on the inherent value of artistic creation and its ability to heal or create cathartic energy, whereas the 'art in therapy' approaches view artistic creation as a tool within a greater therapeutic picture (Madden and Bloom, 2004, p. 140). Within this latter conceptualisation, the arts can be seen as 'one of the tools clinicians have at their disposal for the purposes of diagnosis, prognosis, and treatment' (Belfiore, 2016, p. 13). In this case, artistic elements of combined therapies may help to communicate or reconceptualise notions that are either too painful to verbalise or too complex to describe using the limits of our language but are not deemed to be comprehensive solutions in and of themselves.

This suggests another implicit assumption of the current wellbeing market, which is that, at times, traditional therapies can support an individual's *entire* wellbeing. In contrast, my own experience would suggest that these distinct services, in fact, support different types of wellbeing and that, despite the prioritisation of talking therapies in the marketplace, these too hold as many limitations as artistic provisions. This recognition does not devalue the importance of accessing therapeutic services but prompts a reflection on how power relations can skew our conceptualisation of what quality care looks like and how we should behave as market users.

Participatory Arts (PAs)

Elsewhere in the market, practitioners have shown to be less concerned about the scientific perception of their specialism. Instead, these artists often promote the inherent wellbeing value associated with engagement in the arts. Services like this can be described as Participatory Arts (PAs). By exploring how PAs promote their practices, whilst avoiding the use of specialist job titles, we can gather further insight into the power relations of the marketplace.

Tate (2017) defines PAs as 'a form of art that directly engages the audience in the creative process so that they become participants in the event' (para. 1). These are distinct from traditional forms of engagement with the arts, where audiences are passive viewers and the artist is the bearer of talent. Instead, PAs make space for shared ownership and decision-making, and often exist for the virtue of making rather than the quality of a final product.

PAs differ from formalised therapies, as communities often take part in them for their supportive healing or socialising qualities rather than to resolve a specific trauma. For this reason, PAs are often promoted as preventative measures, distinguishing them from medical provisions which primarily offer responsive care. There is a growing body of literature that advocates for more preventative mental health care, both in the UK (e.g., Knapp, McDaid and Parsonage, 2011; McDaid, Park and Wahlbeck, 2019) and internationally (e.g., Arango et al., 2018; Fusar-Poli et al., 2021). I argue, therefore, that this is a market strength of PAs.

PAs have been used for numerous purposes, but these benefits are often articulated in connection with specific age groups or demographics. Often these demographic boundaries are created within research either to meet the expectations of academic/medical funders, who prefer a succinct and measurable cohort of participants, or to align with policies that prioritise vulnerable demographics. This demonstrates another power dynamic that exists within the Creative Health market, begging the question of whether there are more inclusive methods of measurement available. A risk of using demographics as a basis for research is that the field is not able to evidence its benefits on the general population. Once these services are rolled out on mass, they are in danger of identifying weaknesses too late into the market process, after service-users have already lost trust in the ability of the arts to help them.

Creative Health literature which moves away from demographic labels towards mutual wellbeing needs between participants has, so far, lacked clarity or self-regulation in their definition of terms. This altering of scope leaves them open for criticism about the measurability, replicability, and falsification of their research. One example of this is research into social cohesion. Within this body of literature, researchers have identified that PAs are 'perceived to benefit mental health via improved connectedness; emotional regulation; meaning-making & re-defining identity; and personal growth & empowerment' (O'Donnell, 2021, 15:54:00), however, there are methodological limitations to measuring social cohesion (Gingrich et al., 2020). Likewise, there are various papers on the power of the arts to give voice or empower individuals, but there are axiological issues with how this is defined and measured.

Walsh and Burnett (2021) respond to this by developing theory on 'seeing power' whereby PAs – in this case, filmmaking – can provide participants with the literacy of 'who counts as human, thus whose worldviews are worth knowing' (p. 33) allowing them to negotiate within power structures and maintain their self-worth despite their place within unjust hierarchies. A decolonial project at its heart, this contribution upheld that 'how we know is forged by these power structures, including language, education, and what is valued' (p. 33). By being more specific about the type of voice their research is referring- and responding- to, these authors become exemplary in demonstrating how social investigations can hold rigor and be accountable in their findings. More researchers in the field could benefit from taking this clarity-centred approach to social definitions, as it allows them to advocate for the power of social inquiry, whilst developing outputs that are more inclusive of a range of demographics.

As the field of Creative Health seeks to make PAs more accessible, research has been conducted into barriers to engagement for those who have anxiety or depression (e.g., Fancourt, Baxter and Lorencatto, 2020). This found that people with depression and anxiety are more likely to struggle to engage with PAs due to their psychological and physical capabilities, social opportunities, and both their automatic and reflective motivations to engage. Others who have experienced barriers include people with learning difficulties. Research into this found that 'transport, cost and needing support often got in the way of people being able to go to activities and people needed to feel safe and welcomed when they attend an arts and culture activity' (Gratton, 2020). In the RADIANCE framework, developed at UCL, research has identified over 30 barriers to accessing the arts (*Why is arts engagement uneven? Introducing the RADIANCE Framework*, 2024). This can be used by PA researchers and practitioners to design more accessible and equitable provisions.

By exploring CATs and PAs, I argue that a segregation can be observed, based both on their evaluation protocols and their degree of alignment to the medical model. Brown (2006) describes 'two approaches to visual creativity in mental health care: art therapy, where the emphasis is placed on healing, with the client as patient-to-be-cured; and non-clinical arts activity, where emphasis is placed on art, with the participant as artist-in-the-making' (p. 5). The former seeks to align itself to the medical model of health, relying on training, pre-set outcome measures, and a focus on responsive care (i.e., responding to pre-existing acute mental disorders). The latter, on the other hand, struggles to fit within the medically dominated industry, due in part to the lack of health-based or business-related training undergone by the artists involved.

Through my research, I deduce that PAs primarily record outcomes post-hoc and focus, to a large extent, on preventative care. This has caused some researchers to consider the differences between evidence-based services following a medical model and holistic services which are shaped via user input (e.g., Daykin, 2020, pp. 7–8). An issue which arises from this segregation starts with the public perception of each type of service. Specifically, distinctions of this kind can encourage medical practitioners to treat their artistic counterparts as optional extras, often conceptualising their role as promoting a medical provision rather than offering a provision of their own. As a consequence of this power struggle, an objective of my research is to identify means of promoting service strengths which are inclusive and safe without relying on scientific hierarchies.

Beyond the Market

Without the restrictions of a marketplace, Creative Health is an expansive term – one which describes the way that communities cook together to form bonds and show love, one which appreciates the way that gardening can offer a sense of calm and provide metaphors for growth, and one which acknowledges the importance of creative headspace over the quality or marketability of an artistic output. Creative Health as a movement is inclusive and able to adapt around the unique personalities of different individuals. But place Creative Health into a market and it inevitably becomes shaped by the inequalities that exist within that market system.

Our Creative Health market is shaped by academia – whether it be the gatekeeping of knowledge behind journal paywalls, long-held views of scientific hierarchy over artistic evaluation, or the disproportionate distribution of power between mostly privileged researchers and the grassroots communities they research and speak on behalf of. Our Creative Health market is shaped by capitalism – including the valuing of targeted, pitch-worthy interventions over the holistic, embedded or sustainable outputs, the prioritisation of responsive care (which is easily measured) over preventative care (which is not), and the bias partnerships that form from a network that is highly relational in nature. Finally, our Creative Health market is shaped by medicine – from the ways that members of the public might scrutinise the real value of arts within healthcare, to the way that medications are prioritised over creative provisions even when the evidence is not in their favour, or to the way that the health system attempts to place creative activity into professionalised boxes. We are not unique in needing to battle against the values of a market to protect the values of our movement. However, we can all benefit from holding a greater awareness of how to work within the restraints of a market in a way that ultimately furthers our goals. I hope that through the first section of this book, I have provided information which can support you in this goal.

References

Arango, C. et al. (2018) Preventive strategies for mental health. *The Lancet Psychiatry*, 5(7), pp. 591–604.

Belfiore, E. (2016) The arts and healing: The power of an idea. In: Clift, S. and Camic, P.M. (eds.) *Oxford Textbook of Creative Arts, Health, and Wellbeing: International Perspectives on Practice, Policy, and Research*. Oxford Textbooks in Public Health. Oxford, United Kingdom: Oxford University Press, pp. 11–18.

Brown, L. (2006) *Is Art Therapy? Art for Mental Health at the Millennium*. p. 339. https://www.artsforhealth.org/people/langley-brown-phd-thesis.pdf [Accessed 28/11/2020].

Cohen, J.L., Johnson, J.L. and Orr, P. (eds.) (2015) *Video and Filmmaking as Psychotherapy: Research and Practice*. New York London: Routledge.

Daykin, N. (2020) *Arts, Health and Well-being: A Critical Perspective on Research, Policy and Practice*. Oxon: Routledge.

Dileo, C. and Bradt, J. (2009) On creating the discipline, profession, and evidence in the field of arts and healthcare. *Arts & Health*, 1(2), pp. 168–182.

Fancourt, D., Baxter, L. and Lorencatto, F. (2020) Barriers and enablers to engagement in participatory arts activities amongst individuals with depression and anxiety: Quantitative analyses using a behaviour change framework. *BMC Public Health*, 20(1), p. 272.

Fusar-Poli, P. et al. (2021) Preventive psychiatry: A blueprint for improving the mental health of young people. *World Psychiatry*, 20(2), pp. 200–221.

Gingrich, O.M. et al. (2020) Connections: Participatory art as a factor for social cohesion. In: *Proceedings of EVA London 2020*.

Gratton, N. (2020) People with learning disabilities and access to mainstream arts and culture: A participatory action research approach. *British Journal of Learning Disabilities*, 48(2), pp. 106–114.

Knapp, M., McDaid, D. and Parsonage, M. (2011) Mental health promotion and mental illness prevention: The economic case. [online] HM Government | Department of Health and Social Care. Available at: https://www.gov.uk/government/publications/mental-health-promotion-and-mental-illness-prevention-the-economic-case [Accessed 19/11/2022].

Madden, C. and Bloom, T. (2004) Creativity, health and arts advocacy. *International Journal of Cultural Policy*, 10(2), pp. 133–156.

McDaid, D., Park, A.-L. and Wahlbeck, K. (2019) The economic case for the prevention of mental illness. *Annual Review of Public Health*, 40(1), pp. 373–389.

Mind (2021) *Arts and Creative Therapies*. London: Mind.

O'Donnell, S. (2021) *Development of a participatory arts intervention to promote mental health and wellbeing among men 'at risk' of suicide*. PhD Thesis. Belfast: Queen's University.

Parkinson, C. (2018) *Social Justice, Inequalities, But Arts and Public Health: Weapons of Mass Happiness?* Manchester: Manchester Metropolitan University.

Tate (2017) Participatory Art. *Tate – Art Terms*. Available at: https://www.tate.org.uk/art/art-terms/p/participatory-art [Accessed 29/09/2022].

Walsh, A. and Burnett, S. (2021) 'Seeing power', co-creation and intersectionality in film-making by Ilizwi Lenyaniso Lomhlaba. In: Mkwananzi, F. and Cin, F.M. (eds.) *Post-Conflict Participatory Arts*. London: Routledge, pp. 33–53.

Why Is Arts Engagement Uneven? Introducing the RADIANCE Framework. (2024) Directed by *Why Is Arts Engagement Uneven? Introducing the RADIANCE Framework*. London: UCL.

Part 2

User-Centred Design within Research

Chapter 5

Pragmatism

Using the Market as a Grounding Mechanism within Research

When considering the best methodological approach to use as the basis of my research and framework design, I found myself critiquing many epistemological positions as being too reductive. When we think about mental health and wellbeing, there are aspects that best align with a biomedical perspective, positioning themselves naturally within positivist epistemology, but there are also aspects that are psychosocial, which better position themselves within social constructionist thought. Since my Creative Health Communication Framework aims to be inclusive of all perspectives on mental health and wellbeing, and because I believe that the collective knowledge of mental health and wellbeing is stronger and more insightful than any siloed components, it does not make sense to work within one epistemology at the exclusion of another.

Interrogating this thought further, I wanted to better understand why we necessitate the reductionism of one epistemological basis when human life is a fluid mix of multiple. If it is to make data comparable then other options of comparison are also available. The option that we choose depends on the *purpose* of that comparison. In my case, I want to assist Creative Health professionals in communicating about how their provisions differ from other creative, social, or medical services. In my view, this is better evaluated based on the resonance of a service to the individuals that use it, or the overall value of this service once cost-to-benefit ratios have been considered.

Alternatively, the selection of one epistemological framework may be chosen to indicate a type of truth – an act that ultimately suggests that one form of *truthiness* is more valuable than another. Here I use truthiness to describe 'the quality of seeming or being felt to be true, even if not necessarily true' (Oxford Dictionary Online, 2022). I argue that, within a marketplace, truthiness is more important than *scientia* – that is, 'a type of absolute knowledge of the necessary connections that would explain why certain things are a certain way' (Markie and Folescu, 2021). In a marketplace, service-users are rarely drawn to a provision based on its ability to prove itself undoubtedly true. Rather, they resonate with a form of truthiness that authenticates their humanity, reaches one of their needs, or echoes an aspect of their unique point of view.

DOI: 10.4324/9781003423317-8

For these reasons, I began to search for a different type of epistemology – one that provides an agenda for knowledge prioritisation based on what is useful to a marketplace. This brought me to pragmatism. Pragmatism is an epistemology which posits that the 'meaning of phenomenon derives from its effects on the world, rather than from any intrinsic properties it may have' (Dennis, 2011, p. 464). I believe this makes it particularly compatible to investigations relating to market success, as the *effects* of the market are some of the most influential aspects of modern living.

The Pragmatist Tradition

Pragmatist methodology is born from an understanding that 'the reality of the world is constituted by our practical *orientation* to it' (Williams, 2016, p. 172). In the context of a marketplace, each service-user has a different orientation to the world because they all carry different lived experiences. To design for a marketplace, therefore, involves either the *integration of adaptability* into the service or the *identification of commonality* within a group of service-users' priorities. In the first case, this shifts the focus of research away from a single demographic group towards maximising variation in demographic diversity. In the latter scenario, this shifts the focus of research away from projects that investigate demographics based on inherent characteristics (e.g., the mental health experiences of women), towards common values (e.g., a large portion of women may have mental health challenges relating to gender inequality, but this will not be true for all women, and may also be resonant with people under the trans umbrella, or men with divergent expressions of masculinity).

Important to this conversation is the language of *value perceptions*. These are defined as 'a customer's own perception of a product or service's merit or desirability to them, especially in comparison to a competitor's product' (Kopp, 2020). Relating this back to research and the application of epistemology, I argue that to properly investigate the varied orientations that potential service-users hold in relation to the world, researchers should not seek to challenge the value perceptions identified by service-users. Specifically, I believe that the so-called 'useful data' from service-users' accounts of wellbeing are not simply the identification of need but also the way that they make sense of these needs. Their act of sense-making provides us with insights as to how they might make sense of market offers and this is extremely important if we aspire to succeed within a marketplace or support those that do. Value perceptions affect the way that members of the public engage with services on offer. The goal of our data analysis, therefore, is to identify how health services might satisfy service-users' value-laden needs. This helps us to recognise the importance of communicating these values within needs-centred promotional materials.

Exploring pragmatism further, Peirce (1877, 1878) – often hailed as the father of pragmatism – posited that thoughts engender beliefs. Here, beliefs are defined as *actionable* convictions. Peirce argued that to foster a robust link between *thought* and *action*, doubt must be mitigated through considered investigation (Weaver, 2018, p. 1286). By consulting with potential service-users, I believe we are able to strengthen the connection between this field's knowledge of arts' benefits (the thought) and the market behaviours of service-users (the action). By considering research in these terms, it becomes clearer how we might turn the enthusiasm of our healthcare counterparts into useful action (i.e., the integration of Creative Health services into established healthcare systems or the commissioning of new services outside of these structures). Moreover, through this approach, we hold an opportunity to heighten service-providers' insight into the needs of their service-users and we can influence the way that service-users prioritise and respond to their own needs. This awareness is able to impact both the iterative design of services and their promotion within the marketplace. In a promotional sense, communicating our awareness of nuanced needs to service-users widens the scope for service-providers to succeed, as it builds trust and transparency, and positively manages expectations of their role or offering. In addition, by developing the health literacy of service-users, they are able to become agents of change within a capitalist system, encouraging cultural shifts towards the integration or accessibility of Creative Health provisions. This is a marketplace in action.

Another aspect of pragmatism that is important to address is that it is often considered to be an idealist approach to research, meaning that the parts of the world that it investigates are constructed by the mind. Importantly, when I apply pragmatism to the mental healthcare market, it is the marketplace that I treat as a construct of the mind, rather than mental wellbeing per se. I treat the market as such because it is a man-made system that exists to bring structure to interhuman trade. Our capitalist market is just one structure that could be applied to interhuman trade, so its limitations are contextual to our interaction with capitalist theory. This is important to recognise because many of the inherent tensions that Creative Health providers feel are in relation to the limitations or incompatibility of a capitalist market. I have noticed incidences of creative practitioners talking about their medical or strategic counterparts in an adversarial tone, as if it is their personal values that cause barriers to progression. I believe it is the system that both parties operate in which causes these restrictions. In some incidences, well aligned medical practices may benefit from the capitalist application of healthcare, thus perpetuating the strength of this system. In other scenarios, however, medical practitioners, alike, feel the burden of these restraints. Based on my experience working as a Creative Health Associate at the National Centre for Creative Health, it is the latter of these two scenarios that most often proves to be true. Health partners often *do* share the enthusiasm for bring Creative Health into their systems, but they also refer to the market limitations that are preventing this enthusiasm from turning into action. By recognising the place of a capitalist market, both, in positively and negatively affecting decisions on trade, we bring empathy and understanding into common discussions, and invite more philosophical considerations about the purpose or function of our market and the opportunities or barriers it presents to cultural innovation.

Advantages and Applications of Pragmatism in Creative Health

There are two important advantages that I see when applying pragmatism to the field of Creative Health, some of which impact the context of my Creative Health Communication Framework.

Firstly, Weaver (2018) states that 'taking a pragmatic and balanced or pluralistic position [within research] will help improve communication among researchers from different paradigms' (p. 1288). I believe that this is particularly useful for the Creative Health movement, as it deals with stakeholders that typically work from polarised methodologies (Su and Colander, 2013). This has many useful applications across the field of Creative Health and will ultimately be instrumental in our growth. Applying this specifically to my Creative Health Communication Framework, it can now be used within collaborations and debates. In this sense, it has been birthed from a pluralistic stance and has also become a tool to foster more pluralistic work within future collaborations. Adding to this, since the framework does not prioritise one epistemological basis over another it can, in theory, encourage service-providers to focus on the *practical* outcomes of their services, as felt by their service-users.

Secondly, I invite you to consider the status quo of evaluation procedures within healthcare. The safeguarding of service-users has rightfully been prioritised and this can necessitate an understanding (evaluation) of a service's ability to cause harm or healing. However, there is also a safeguarding concern attached to ill-fitting or oversaturated evaluation procedures. For many creative, cultural, and heritage practitioners, the act of evaluating provisions using outdated or misaligned evaluation tools can leave them feeling disenfranchised, misunderstood, and saddened by the way this negatively affects the person-centredness of their provisions. The act of forcibly evaluating wellbeing outcomes can ultimately lead to feedback fatigue in service-users, which can reduce or counteract the positive outcomes of engaging in a service. By looking at this through a pragmatist lens, we can make this conflict of intent more visible. Consequently, we can consider the best way to respond in scenarios where service-user satisfaction is high, but chances to evaluate in a meaningfully way are low or at the detriment to the service's benefits. I advocate that service-providers be offered more flexibility to communicate in terms of the needs they perceive their services to fulfil, for either their service-users or their funders, rather than just the ability of these services to be measured in a controlled environment. These holistic and adaptable outcomes can be observed by service-providers on a daily basis and can often, therefore, be communicated more effectively via their personal insights and tailored design choices. The need for a Creative Health Communication Framework, in this context, is to strengthen the sophistication of this communication and encourage observation of the intricacies of their offering (i.e., their unique selling points/means of differentiation). This will contribute towards providing confidence to funders that the service-provider doesn't, simply, have good intent, but that their intent has been meaningfully dissected, designed around, and monitored in its application.

The Dangers of Assimilating with Market Interests

Whilst I am a big advocate for pragmatism as a tool for innovation and service-user satisfaction, it is not without its limitations. This is true of any epistemology. As I invite you to apply a pragmatic viewpoint to your own research and practice, it becomes important to consider the downsides of this framing. Here I discuss two areas that I am particularly aware of.

Firstly, for some artistic practitioners, the idea of assimilating their practices to the philosophies of a capitalist economy may cause discomfort. In this case, I argue that once assimilative power is afforded to Creative Health service-providers, they are granted more opportunity to rebel against other misalignments of the market system and can seek to shift cultural norms/power relations in the long term. Importantly, I believe it is only once the outputs of artistic care are more evenly distributed, across systems and geographies, that cross-disciplinary providers can have fair discussions. The current landscape, in comparison, is made up of system insiders and outsiders. During this period, when artistic providers are considered outsiders, they will continue to hold less market power than their counterparts – even those who hold comparable skills, knowledge, and expertise. Once fairer collaboration spaces have been fostered, and if approached mindfully, this could give rise to conversations which can pick apart and interrogate the hierarchical effectiveness of different provisions, based on newly evidenced successes and limitations, rather than relying on outdated or philosophically-led biases. I understand this as a positive consequence of pragmatism, but I am sensitive to the ethical issues of drawing disempowered value-sets towards the behaviours of dominant power systems – that is, asking artists to reconceptualise their outputs in market terms. Esposito and Evans-Winters (2021) highlight that using the tools of oppressive systems of power rarely emancipates voices which are silenced by this system. There is a lot of truth in this claim, so despite my intentions of levelling-out power structures and removing artists from the shackles of hierarchies-of-knowledge, this is an important barrier of pragmatism to consider when applying to your own work.

Secondly, my interest in the way that researchers read or apply data from participants – in relation to value perceptions – carries an inherent emphasis on patient-centred care. Importantly, in my application of pragmatism, this patient-centred care falls short of Todres, Dahlberg and Galvin's (2007) 'lifeworld-led care,' which promotes a movement away from 'patients as consumers (an economic emphasis) or patients as citizens (a political emphasis)' (Galvin and Todres, 2013, p. 36). There are many merits to their approach, and for Creative Health advocates who are interested in catalysing political or cultural change at a system-wide level, this might be more appropriate. In the case of pragmatist inquiry that is focused on service success within the current marketplace, however, the lenses of consumers and citizens are necessary, as consumerist and citizen behaviours provide instrumental context about how to improve the design of – and communication about – Creative Health services. For different researchers or practitioners, there will be different intent in terms of either shifting the culture of a market to be more habitable in the long term or finding a means of survival within the marketplace as it stands. It will be vital that this intent is considered and discussed within collaborative teams, in the early stages of project conceptualisation and design, to aid cohesion and to avoid conflict further into the project.

Applications of Pragmatism: Design Theory

The study of services in a marketplace can be done in one of two directions. In a bottom-up approach, the research begins with a pre-identified service and stakeholders then investigate the market with the intention of finding a place where their service can sit within it (Figure 5.1). Alternatively, a top-down approach means that the research begins at the level of the macroeconomy to identify gaps in the market that services could be designed to fill.

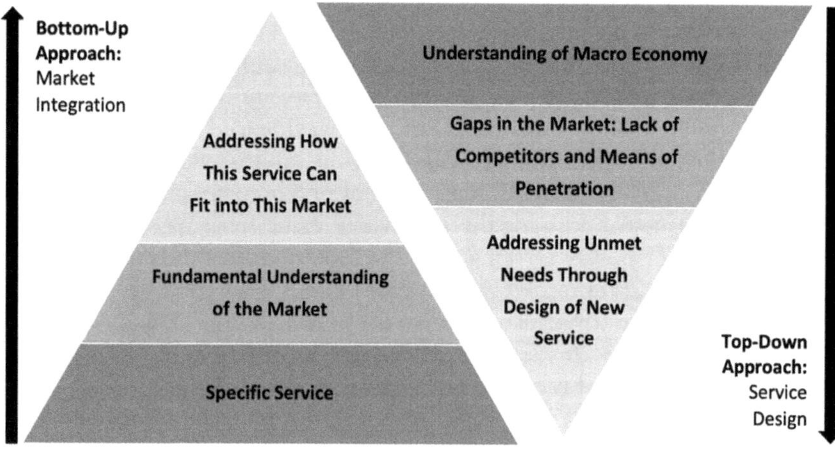

Figure 5.1 Diagram illustrating the difference between a bottom-up approach to design and a top-down approach to design. Here 'bottom' refers to a single service-provider and 'top' refers to the macro marketplace.

The first approach centres the service as the constant and seeks to align it with the most relevant service-user needs available. Consideration of whether another service can meet these needs more effectively is done simply to strengthen the competitiveness of service promotion or adapting elements of future service design. The second approach, on the other hand, considers the needs of service-users first and then designs services around these requirements. Theoretically, this approach should produce services that consider user needs more thoroughly and are, therefore, designed for optimal function. Here, the strengths of other services are considered with the intention of ensuring that new service design fulfils new functions and that, consequently, the market is working more effectively.

A bottom-up approach to market interaction is often used by service-providers who favour the Minimum Viable Product (MVP) model of marketing. This model encourages businesses to get their provision to market quickly, despite known/potential design flaws, to achieve profits as soon as possible. The model allows for in-market innovation and a service is improved using ongoing user feedback; however, this innovation is only prioritised in cases where greater profits can be achieved. The top-down approach, on the other hand, prioritises quality service over short-term profitability. This model proposes that by meeting the needs of a user more meaningfully, market power can be derived in the long term through quality assurance and brand reputation.

In my work, I prioritise a top-down approach to market interaction as it is more readily able to provide insight to *numerous* service-providers. By starting with the strengths and weaknesses of the economic context, I can improve the effectiveness of the Creative Health market by promoting a more comprehensive range of care.

Service-providers reading this book may have already designed services, as seen in the bottom-up approach. I argue that since Creative Health services lack power within the market, it is entirely possible that they are already serving some of these unmet needs but have not been able to communicate them in a manner that draws in funding or inspires interaction of service-users. In this case, their approach can differ from the approach prioritised in my work, whilst remaining aligned to my wider goals.

There is a second way that I differ from individual researchers or service-providers in my application of design theory – namely in the diamond pattern I am following.

Created by The Design Council in 2004, the *Double Diamond Design Process* describes the visual pattern created through a divergence and convergence strategy (Design Council, 2023). Here, divergence describes the widening of opportunity through new knowledge or ideas, and convergence denotes the act of filtering this knowledge for a specific purpose or prioritised outcome. In the Double Diamond Design Process, two sets of divergence and convergence occur (Figure 5.2). In the first set, service-designers collect a

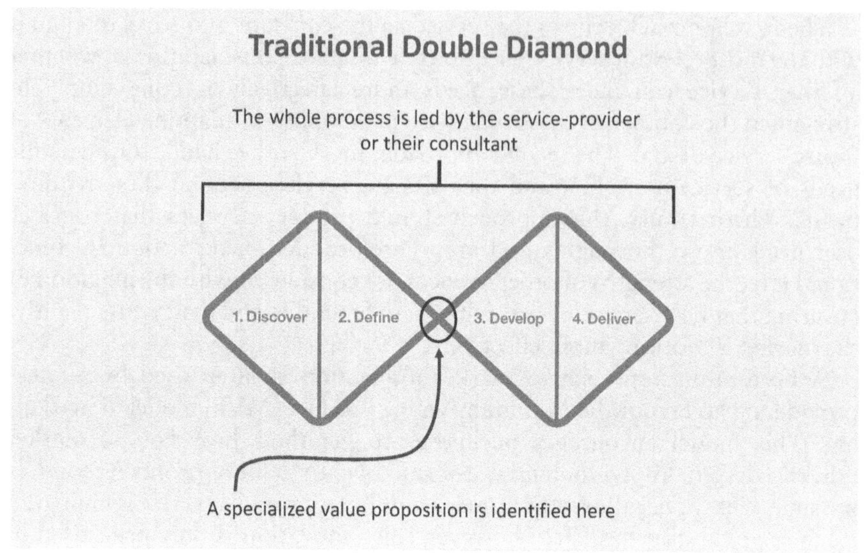

Figure 5.2 The Double Diamond Design Process – designed by the Design Council, Copyright of Design Council, sharable via CC BY 4.0 license, reproduced for illustrative purposes only. Labels added by Dr Jane Hearst to compare against the Modified Double Diamond Design Process (Figure 5.3). Original content and license notice available from: https://www.designcouncil.org.uk/our-resources/the-double-diamond/.

wide scope of information about service-users, then filter the information into defining patterns. In the second set, this information is then used to develop unrestricted ideas to solve service-user needs, followed by a filtering of ideas into pragmatic solutions (Design Council and Technology Strategy Board, 2015). These stages align to the IDEO Human Centred Design Toolkit, which describes a journey from concrete observations, and their associated stories, towards abstract themes, and then a movement from abstract opportunities and solutions towards concrete prototypes with a clear implementation plan (Barnes and Du Preez, 2015; IDEO, 2015).

Since the function of the original Double Diamond Design Process was created to be used by individual service-providers, and focus on a single value proposition (i.e., service-user need), I needed to adapt its design towards the function of a market researcher (Figure 5.3).

By modifying the purpose of this model to inform the enterprise development of external parties (i.e., Creative Health researchers and practitioners other than myself) – whereby my role is to support a sector rather than a single organisation – I argue that my modified Double Diamond Design Process makes a more comprehensive use of service-user data. Where, in the original Double Diamond Design Process, much of the valuable data and

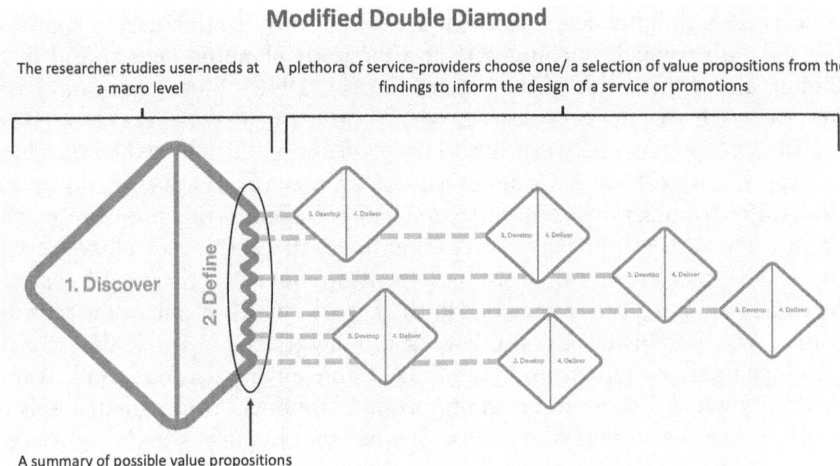

Figure 5.3 Hearst's modified version of The Double Diamond Design Process – originally version designed by The Design Council..Original content and license notice available from: https://www.designcouncil.org.uk/our-resources/the-double-diamond/.

opportunities identified along the way are naturally excluded from the final service design (i.e., that which did not align with an organisation's strengths), the modified Double Diamond Design Process widens the scope of who can use this data to inform the improvement of their provisions.

My modified Double Diamond Design Process demonstrates the power that comes from introducing a researcher into the first half of the design process. Specifically, it allows findings to be utilised by a range of service-providers and, therefore, optimises the impact that these findings can have on the industry. Following the process of this modified model, I identified a breadth of service-user values and then created a framework tool to make sense of these. Relevant portions of this information can be extracted by different service-providers and can be applied within services or promotions to make them more specific, transparent, and market-driven.

Final Thoughts...

As this chapter has explored, the Pragmatism Interpretive Framework suggests that 'value can only be determined by practical application and consequences' (O'Leary, 2007). Consequently, the magnitude of success gained through a pragmatist research project is measured by how much the information collected can inform practical action.

As we move towards the next chapter of the book, I wanted to draw your attention to one final consideration. I believe that pragmatic intent is well aligned to the practice of action research (McNiff, 2017) since both are concerned with influencing practical action. Action research uses 'a spiral of steps, each of which is composed of a circle of planning, action and fact-finding about the result of the action' (Lewin, 1946). I am a big fan of the iterative nature of action research, which is one of the reasons I fostered an iterative negotiation between lived and professional insights when developing my Creative Health Communication Framework. However, my work does differ from action research, as *the action* linked to this project (i.e., the application of the framework) has taken place after my research was complete. The success of my work is dependent on researchers and service-providers applying the framework to their work, which is one of the reasons I invite you to consider the framework as emergent. It is a tool that can be developed and altered around the needs of an evolving market, and it is this flexibility which I deem to be an important component of pragmatist epistemology. In a world that is not static, neither should our research knowledge nor practical outputs be.

References

Barnes, V. and Du Preez, V. (2015) Mapping empathy and ethics in the design process. In: *7th International DEFSA Conference*, Design Education Forum of Southern Africa. Available at: http://digitalknowledge.cput.ac.za/bitstream/11189/5927/1/Barnes_Veronica_du%20Preez_Vikki_FID_2015.pdf (Accessed 27/10/2020).

Dennis, A. (2011) Pragmatism and symbolic interactionism. In: Jarvie, I. and Zamora-Bonilla, J. (eds.) *The SAGE Handbook of the Philosophy of Social Sciences.* 1 Oliver's Yard, 55 City Road, London EC1Y 1SP. United Kingdom: SAGE Publications Ltd, pp. 463–474. Available at: https://doi.org/10.4135/9781473913868.n24

Design Council (2023) The Double Diamond: A universally accepted depiction of the design process. *Design Council: Our Resources*, 11 May. Available at: https://www.designcouncil.org.uk/our-resources/the-double-diamond/ (Accessed 31/10/2024).

Design Council and Technology Strategy Board (2015) *Design Methods for Developing Services: An Introduction to Service Design and a Selection of Service Design Tools.* Available at: https://www.designcouncil.org.uk/sites/default/files/asset/document/Design%20methods%20for%20developing%20services.pdf (Accessed 27/10/2020).

Esposito, J. and Evans-Winters, V.E. (2021) *Introduction to Intersectional Qualitative Research.* 1st Edition. Thousand Oaks: SAGE Publications, Inc.

Galvin, K. and Todres, L. (2013) *Caring and Well-being: A Lifeworld Approach.* Routledge. Available at: https://doi.org/10.4324/9780203082898

IDEO (ed.) (2015) *The Field Guide to Human-centered Design: Design Kit.* 1st Edition. San Francisco, Calif: IDEO.

Kopp, C.M. (2020) Perceived value explained: What it is, why it's important. *Investopedia*, 30 November. Available at: https://www.investopedia.com/terms/p/perceived-value.asp (Accessed 18/06/2021).

Lewin, K. (1946) Action research and minority problems. *Journal of Social Issues*, 2(4), pp. 34–46. Available at: https://doi.org/10.1111/j.1540-4560.1946.tb02295.x

Markie, P. and Folescu, M. (2021) Rationalism vs. empiricism. *Stanford Encyclopedia of Philosophy*, 2 September. Available at: https://plato.stanford.edu/entries/rationalism-empiricism/ (Accessed 15/03/2024).

McNiff, J. (2017) *Action Research: All You Need to Know*. 1st Edition. Thousand Oaks, CA: SAGE Publications.

O'Leary, Z. (2007) *The Social Science Jargon Buster*. 1 Oliver's Yard, 55 City Road, London England EC1Y 1SP. United Kingdom: SAGE Publications Ltd. Available at: https://doi.org/10.4135/9780857020147

Oxford Dictionary Online (2022) Truthiness.

Peirce, C.S. (1877) The fixation of belief. *Popular Science Monthly*, 12(1), pp. 1–15.

Peirce, C.S. (1878) How to make our ideas clear. *Popular Science Monthly*, 12(2), pp. 286–302.

Su, H. and Colander, D. (2013) A failure to communicate: The fact-value divide and the Putnam-Dasgupta debate. *Erasmus Journal for Philosophy and Economics*, 6(2), p. 1. Available at: https://doi.org/10.23941/ejpe.v6i2.131

Todres, L., Galvin, K. and Dahlberg, K. (2007) Lifeworld-led healthcare: Revisiting a humanising philosophy that integrates emerging trends. *Medicine, Health Care and Philosophy*, 10(1), pp. 53–63. Available at: https://doi.org/10.1007/s11019-006-9012-8

Weaver, K. (2018) Pragmatic Paradigm. In: Frey, B.B. (ed.) *The Sage Encyclopedia of Educational Research, Measurement, and Evaluation*. Los Angeles: SAGE Reference.

Williams, M. (2016) *Key Concepts in the Philosophy of Social Research*. Los Angeles: SAGE (SAGE key concepts).

Chapter 6

Critical Psychology

Wellbeing at the Intersection of the Individual and the Market

Introduction

When discussing or piloting the Creative Health Communication Framework with others, one of the most frequent questions I get asked is why I chose to include combative language like 'threats to wellbeing.' At the heart of my answer is an awareness that the way we experience mental health and wellbeing at the individual level is different to how we are taught to conceptualise mental health and wellbeing as a society. The communication style that I promote in my framework is not the only option available to Creative Health advocates – that is the nature of language and, for some, other communication options may be a better fit. What my framework does offer, however, is an acknowledgement of the prevalence of capitalist influence in our lives – a way of thinking that communicates in terms of resources, exchanges, value negotiation, having/not having, giving, and taking. By being aware of this, and how it positively or negatively affects our conceptualisation and management of mental health and wellbeing, my framing is both reminiscent of how mental health and wellbeing is discussed in medical circles, whilst holding space for growth, nuance, and greater person-centredness in its application.

In this chapter, I explore some of the theory around the negotiation space that exists between the individual and a capitalist marketplace. Specifically, this involves the exploration of critical psychology and its effects on phenomenology.

Consciousness in Context

Phenomenology, as it was originally conceived, involved the study of pure consciousness and the meanings of a transcendental ego. Modern phenomenology, on the other hand, has shifted towards the study of consciousness and meaning in context.

My research interests look at how we experience and make sense of mental health and wellbeing, so consciousness and meaning-making are key to my work. When I consider what context needs to be acknowledged and

DOI: 10.4324/9781003423317-9

interrogated in my work, I am acutely aware of capitalism, marketplaces, and their effects on how we think in society. Consequently, I believe that understanding the context of the marketplace is important to understanding how mental health and wellbeing are experienced in a capitalist society.

To offer an example, colonised conceptualisations of wellbeing affect the public's day-to-day language. Specifically, western psychology has long encouraged a structuralist approach to vocalising wellbeing. This includes ideas like Freud's layered person, consisting of the super-ego, ego, and id. These theories have penetrated into our daily lives, as citizens of western cultures frequently talk of people in layered metaphors such as being 'like an onion,' 'digging deep,' and 'the core self.' These metaphors are not necessarily wrong, but they represent just one view of wellbeing (Hayward, 2022). Other cultures do not carry these structured concepts, and this should not make their contributions any less valuable to this project.

Other types of structuralist language, which I have chosen to take a neutral stance on, include the language of psychological *needs*. To talk in terms of 'need' theorises that every individual's wellbeing shares similarities in the basic resources they require to survive. The concept of psychological needs emerged in 1927 in response to growing consensus over physiological needs (Hayward, 2022). It could be argued that physiological needs have a clearer correlation – for example, you cannot *survive* without water, whereas it might be more accurate to say you simply cannot *thrive* without autonomy, competence, and relatedness – the three psychological needs referenced in Self-Determination Theory (Deci and Ryan, 1985).

In places, throughout this book, I too use the language of need. However, I have tried to balance this by using the language of non-structuralist approaches, such as Narrative Therapy, which replaces *needs* with words such as *wants*, *hopes*, and *likes*. This language attempts to decentre the therapist or service-provider from an individual'/service-user's experience. Narrative Therapists posit that the wording of 'needs' is often used by people who consider themselves specialists of mental health and wellbeing. Consequently, they can suppose that they can understand aspects of an individual's experience better than the individual themselves – such as their deeper layers of consciousness or functions of their brain. Comparatively, wants, hopes, and likes feel more intimately connected to the individual, which affords them power to challenge any of the providers' preconceptions that do not resonate with them (Hayward, 2022). This positively reenforces the importance of service-user knowledge sets and the expertise of live experience.

What I want to argue throughout this chapter is that providers are not wrong to use this language – with the consent of those they support – but we must understand why we use it, what we exclude in the normalisation of this language, and how we hold ourselves to account. This is where critical psychology comes in.

> Critical psychologists look at trends in psychology and psychotherapy with an eye toward how they either support the status quo or empower people. They are concerned with the way our society is psychologized and how Western psychological ideas are exported around the world.
>
> (Holzman, 2014)

In the context of this discussion, a Critical Psychology lens involves an awareness of how dominant concepts of wellbeing and mental healthcare might, in fact, repress or delegitimise the views of minoritised groups.

An example of academic thought that holds undertones of Critical Psychology is Greco and Stenner (2013). They dispute traditional psychological theory that equates positive mental state with happiness, whereby happiness 'is precisely the feature of splitting the subject from their world; of treating feelings and desires as purely internal, individual and subjective affairs' (p. 1). Instead, Greco and Stenner encourage the pursuit of joy – defined as 'the embodied connection between self and world' (p. 1). They make a value judgement that wellbeing provisions within a market are good when they allow a service-user to embody joy. This is a very different notion from historical markets which have focused on the ability of the service-user to *survive* through negative mental health experiences rather than *flourish* through positive mental wellbeing experiences.

The Lifeworld Approach

The relationship between a service-user's whole wellbeing experience and the portion of wellbeing that a practitioner supports links to Husserl's (1936) lifeworld approach to phenomenology. Galvin and Todres (2013) explain that this approach describes the lifeworld as 'the beginning place-flow from which we divide up our experiences into more abstract categories and names' (p. 25). They go on to suggest that 'without understanding the fullness of these qualitative dimensions, health care systems and practices may become overly concerned with partial goals and issues that measure quality in ways that are superficial and even potentially dehumanising' (p. 26).

My understanding of the lifeworld is that it extends past the feelings or moods we might associate with wellbeing, into the environments we access, the stories we tell, the social connections we share, and many other contextual factors that shape our wellbeing from moment to moment. This context shapes both our experience of wellbeing and our understanding of what it encapsulates. To use a metaphor: imagine a single moment in time, captured in a photograph. We can describe the specific state that might be deduced from that photo, detached from time and narrative. But all that description tells us is the mood elicited in that photographic moment. Whereas, take that same moment and situate it within a series of photographs, and we begin to get a more nuanced understanding of a wellbeing system and how diverse the scope of wellbeing experiences are within this system. Turn that collection of photographs into a film reel and suddenly we have given temporal context to these diverse moments. This allows us to appreciate the space between moments, such as what factors lead towards a transformation of mood and wellbeing, how long those transformations take to change, and how many of the co-existing emotions shift within that transformation. We can register the direction of mood from good to bad or bad to good, and develop a better appreciation of how negative moments can belong in a narrative of positivity, and vice versa.

In this conceptualisation of wellbeing, our definition of wellbeing is ever-changing and dynamic. For this reason, the 'truth' of what wellbeing is, is not static either. This is why researchers like Kara (2015) propose a return to 'the view of the polymaths: that knowledge is worth having, no matter where it originates, and the more diverse a person's knowledge, the more likely they will be able to identify and implement creative solutions to problems' (p. 21). For this reason, both people with lived experience of a phenomena and those who come from diverse professional backgrounds become crucial voices in the design and implementation of wellbeing services. Collectively they offer us a more comprehensive view of wellbeing, a broader definition and scope. Only with this broader understanding can we get close to appreciating what the lifeworld of wellbeing may contain in its fullness. Galvin and Todres (2013) argue that such descriptions of wellbeing incorporate pathologised descriptions of the body whilst also expanding beyond this to record how that body meaningfully functions within the world (p. 29). This is a more complete understanding of wellbeing as it captures 'the interaction of health and illness-related phenomena with individuals' holistic and interrelated experiences of meaning' (p. 30).

Practically, the way that researchers and practitioners can balance the wholeness of the lifeworld with the specifics of their research or service delivery is through cylindrical/iterative forms of knowledge generation – both of which align closely with the epistemological underpinnings of pragmatism and design theory, explored in the previous chapter of this book.

Dewey's (1902–1944) contribution to pragmatism focused on the cylindrical/iterative relationship between beliefs and actions, in which 'beliefs arise from our prior actions and the outcomes of our actions are found in our beliefs' (Morgan, 2014, p. 1046). This mirrors the ideology underpinning design theory; an equally iterative approach used to turn needs into solutions and then use the outcomes of solutions to gain a clearer understanding of needs (Martin, 2009; Brown and Katz, 2009; Tschimmel, 2012). Where this relationship can also be found is within hermeneutic phenomenology. Hans-Georg Gadamer (1975) developed the 'hermeneutic circle' (Keane, 2016, pp. 299–311) which suggests that each time a study returns to view the whole there should be a re-conceptualisation of what the whole is, informed by the new information learnt via an individual's experience, rather than a return to an a priori whole. This is the type of pragmatic application of the hermeneutic circle that I promote when researching or designing around wellbeing. Here, the whole is the lifeworld of wellbeing, and focused information can include market forces or individual experiences depending on the goal of research or design.

Schön (1983) maintained that application of the hermeneutic circle within design involves defining the whole as a 'conversation with the situation' (pp. 76–104). It is through this dialectic movement between the part and the whole that the 'paradoxical problem of needing to know part of something in order to know the whole, but to know the whole we must come to know the part' (Williams, 2016, p. 99) can be overcome. Even more importantly, the use of this technique has been shown to be instrumental in breaking down the communication barriers that exist between medical practitioners and healthcare service-users (Toombs, 1987). This in turn has contributed towards reducing the frictions that exist between pathologized and holistic providers of care – an outcome I am keen to replicate and promote in my work.

Moreover, unlike a descriptive phenomenological approach – where participant knowledge is presented entirely as it was delivered by participants – the hermeneutic approach encourages researchers to be purpose-driven. In my case, the purpose of this book is to unveil opportunities for language development and better service design in the Creative Health movement. Such language can break down participants' experiences into manageable and promotable pieces, whilst recognising the wholeness of their experience and supporting multi-modal care responses.

Critical Theory

Earlier in this book, I outlined the logic behind prioritising the market as a grounding mechanism. This logic stressed that it is the market that affords power whereas competitors, such as mental health providers from the field of medicine, are simply afforded power due to their compatibility with the market. In this chapter, I have asserted that it is ethically advantageous to incorporate service-users' voices into the investigation, due to their insight into the lifeworld of wellbeing. However, service-user voices and market voices also compete in power negotiations, whereby the market is often the dominant player.

As I considered an appropriate way to align to the market, it was ethically important to make explicit where the limits to service-users' influence lie. To illustrate this, I have built upon Habermas' articulation of Critical Social Theory (Habermas, 1968; Baynes, 2016; Jackson, 2017) to visualise where, in my work, wellbeing is positioned between service-users and the market, and why, therefore, it is important to differentiate market wellbeing from a more essentialist form of holistic wellbeing.

Critical Social Theory is a field of research which describes the relationship between an individual/demographic and a system of power. Within this book, I am interested in the relationship between a service-user's lifeworld and the wellbeing market that they access support through (Figure 6.1). I propose that the in-between space – between the whole unique experience of wellbeing known to a service-user and the various forces of the market, such as the conceptualisation of wellbeing understood by individual service-providers – is a space of compromise and equilibrium. This space represents the collaborative conceptualisation of wellbeing that is built during a market transaction, whereby the limitations of the market are applied on top of a wellbeing experience and compatible needs/support systems are identified within these limitations. This means that the needs that are responded to are not necessarily those that matter most to the service-user, in the absence of market resources in that area, nor do they align entirely to the theoretical idea that a service-provider had for their service ahead of adapting it around a real human. Within this logic, a service-provider becomes a facilitator of the user-market

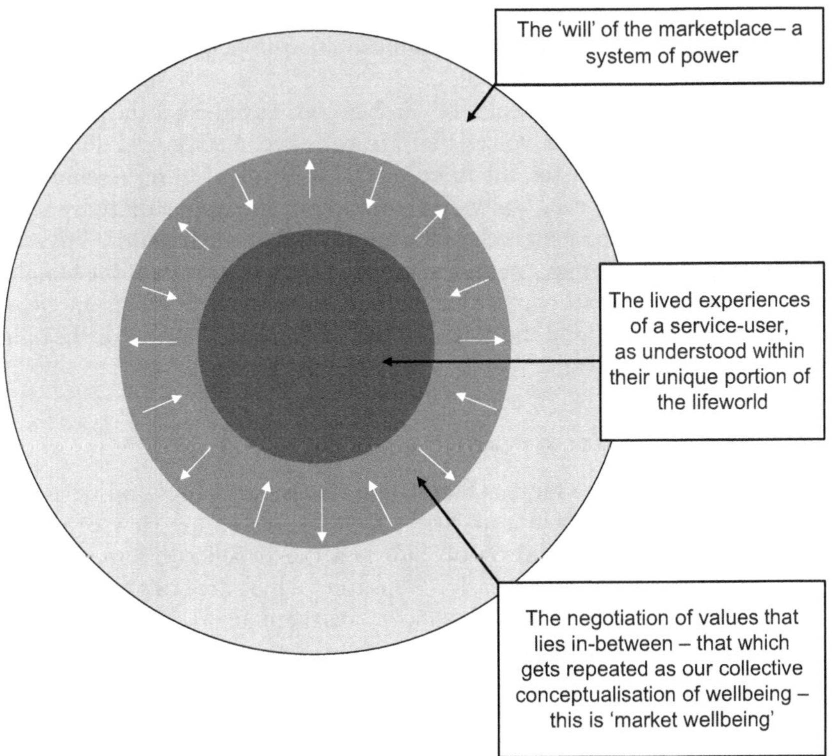

Figure 6.1 Visualisation of the relationship between a service-user's lifeworld and the wellbeing market that they access support through.

relationship; amplifying the benefits of services for their users whilst operating within the confines of the market's philosophical limitations.

By developing Critical Social Theory in this way, I make explicit how the themes of this book necessitate a definition of wellbeing that is neither the unwavering truth sought by the sciences nor the idealistic goal of many artists and market-sceptics. The former does not acknowledge the wholeness of the individual and their lifeworld – simply the parts of the market (either resources or philosophy) that prioritise the pursuit of truth and targeted intervention. The latter does not acknowledge the limitations of the market – simply the idealistic view of how we would respond to the lifeworld if it could be known in its fullness and not be shaped by market forces.

By clarifying the difference between service-user conceptualisations of wellbeing and those held by systems such as the medical sciences and the healthcare market, this project acknowledges two important things. Firstly, these two concepts are not mutually exclusive and thus do not benefit from being placed within a hierarchy of knowledge. Secondly, the findings of a research project are particularly relevant to the market that exists at the time of data collection and will, therefore, need to be built upon in the future as the market shifts and new types of philosophies/modes of delivery/promotional language become important.

As the body of Creative Health research grows, I argue that the greater the variety of service-provider voices that are collected, heard, and allowed to shape the market wellbeing, the more service-users can feel represented and included. In this case, each individual could have the opportunity to access better alignment in their market wellbeing (the space between the lifeworld and the market). Here they could develop their own unique relationship with the services, rather than conforming to one dominant theoretical model of wellbeing designed around the majority, western cultural norms, or the opinions of privileged scholars.

The Language of Resources

Much of this chapter, so far, has focused on theoretical lenses and what they teach us about wellbeing in a market. I have expressed my view of what a more equitable market might look like and the benefits this might hold. However, there are limitations to decolonisation which are born from embedded language structures. For example, marketplace language such as 'resources' and 'assets' have been normalised into western discussions of wellbeing (Hayward, 2022). I believe it is this language framework that has led much of us in the west to talk in terms of 'resilience' when discussing wellbeing. To better understand how we commonly use this language and what limiting effects it has on our view of the lifeworld, I finish with a discussion on resilience theory. I include this here as an example of how one aspect of market wellbeing can be explored more closely, whilst still considering the whole – thereby offering an example of how the hermeneutic circle can be applied in practice.

Masten (2014) proposes that resilience 'can be broadly defined as the capacity of a dynamic system to adapt successfully to disturbances that threaten system function, viability, or development' (p. 6). My observations suggest that the theoretical model of *Engineering Resilience* informs the most common understandings of resilience in the public eye. Engineering Resilience focuses on how stable a system is – in our case, a wellbeing system – and how well it aligns with ideal conditions. This approach assumes there *is* one best version of the system, similar to what you might find in an engineering project. It uses clear methods to enhance system resources when facing known challenges. (Angeler and Allen, 2016, p. 618).

Key terms in this type of resilience are resiliency, return time/recovery, and resistance. Resiliency is the system's ability to bounce back. Return time/recovery measures how quickly this happens, and resistance describes the system's ability to withstand change. (Angeler and Allen, 2016, pp. 618–619).

For essentialist researchers or structural psychology practitioners, this style of resilience may accurately describe their relationship with wellbeing goals. Social constructivists, however, may suggest that this type of resilience – one that is designed around manufactured structures – is far too simple to be applied to human wellbeing or ever-changing lifeworlds. These lead to the question: should we remove the focus on resilience in that case?

As you will later see in my Creative Health Communication Framework, I have chosen to embrace these structuralist elements of language, not because they are the most productive way of describing wellbeing for every person, but because they align experiences of wellbeing to the markets 'way of knowing.' I agree with the social constructivist notions that Engineering Resilience is too limiting a structure to be applied to the lifeworld. However, I also believe that real change happens in the negotiation space between a lifeworld and a system of power – as described earlier in this chapter. The language of resources is one that both the public and the marketplace can share, so I am hesitant to push for its removal from our conversations. Instead, I look for alternative models of resilience. One's which can align to the language of a marketplace without limiting the lifeworld in the way that Engineering Resilience may. This is where Ecological Resilience comes in.

Alternative Models of Resilience

Ecological Resilience offers a more dynamic conceptualisation of resilience, as it is designed around the complexity of natural systems. Quinlan et al. (2016) comment that, Ecological Resilience 'assumes that a system has multiple alternate equilibrium and focuses on the capacity of a system to maintain, including through reorganisation, its essential structure and function when confronted with shocks' (p. 2). Applying this to the lifeworld, I suggest that at any living moment a human only interacts with a portion of what their lifeworld could be. For example, in a different market, individuals would likely experience wellbeing in very different ways to how they experience in our current marketplace because the way that their wellbeing experience would be described and compared to other systems, or the resources and pressures that they interacted with, would be different. We know, therefore, that humans are capable of adaptation. Where resources are abundant and social rhetoric is complementary to our goals, we can apply these resources based on compatibility or desire. Likewise, when resources are scarce and social rhetoric attempts to discredit our chosen modes of maintaining wellbeing, we are able to innovate, challenge the status quo, find our allies, and thrive despite opposition. Ecological Resilience is the framework that allows us to see this latter scenario as a possibility.

Key terms used in Ecological Resilience include adaptive capacity, cross-scale resilience, and functional diversity. Here, adaptive capacity describes the flexibility of a system. Cross-scale resilience indicates measurement both within and across a range of factors. Functional diversity focuses on the variety of roles organisms play in communities and ecosystems (Angeler and Allen, 2016, pp. 618–619).

Crucially, the rhetoric within Creative Health literature around positive wellbeing indicates that advocates of the arts typically conceptualise resilience as a complex (and therefore ecological) system. For example, Hanlon and Carlisle (2016) state that they 'understand the world both as a resource to be used and a complex machine that needs managing' (p. 21). Research also indicates that creativity is a useful tool in nurturing complex resilience systems. In the next chapter, I will look at the place of narrative in humans' ability to renew their sense of self and change the state of their wellbeing, centring the narration of the individual along the way. This nicely compliments the writing of Quinlan et al. (2016) who describe self-organization as 'a key aspect of complex adaptive systems that enables them to regenerate and transform' (p. 2).

Beyond Resilience

Looking at the theory of resilience more critically, I find that, whilst the rhetoric around resilience can help us understand how individuals relate to the world around them, it doesn't capture the complete picture. Namely, his framing posits that it is the sole responsibility of the individual to improve and adapt. Conversely, Ungar (2018) contends

> 'when considering resilience in communities [...] an analysis of power relations (historic and present) must also be made. The division of structural power shapes the capacity of any individual or group accessing and employing resources'.
>
> (p. 34)

MacKinnon and Derickson's (2013) critique of resilience theory builds on this, by reasoning that resilience rhetoric places the responsibility of wellbeing maintenance on the individual. They proclaim that this is unjust as it ignores the influence of systematic inequalities, the economic system of capitalism that relies on these inequalities, and discriminative government policies that prioritise the market over the social (pp. 258–267). Critically they argue that 'resources of instability and crisis that affect urban and regional economies can be seen as internal to capitalism as a system, rather than as immutable external forces to which local groups and communities must continually adapt' (p. 261).

With this in mind, service-providers working in Creative Health may wish to consider who they are attempting to influence through their provisions. Whether that be a service-user who is trying to develop resilience, an influential stakeholder who has the power to reduce external pressure on the individual, or a complex mix of the two. MacKinnon and Derickson (2013) propose that the best way to shift away from resilience as the archetypal response to negative wellbeing, is by updating the language towards resourcefulness (pp. 263–266). This language captures the individual's experience more holistically, by acknowledging both their management of and access to resources (p. 263). What I think is powerful about this theoretical model is that it continues to use market language – of resources and exchange – but through the lens of equity and power. Here, resources refer not only to internal strengths, but also external materials, social power relations, skillsets, and technical knowledge – the core features of a market itself!

Final Thoughts...

To conclude this chapter, I leave you with a final metaphor.

Let us compare the abstraction of 'wellbeing' to that of a garden. For different people their idea of a perfect garden is vastly different. One person may prefer a garden full of lush and varied plants, attracting birds and bees to provide tranquillity, whereas another person might prefer a garden that is less nature-heavy, so that it becomes easier to maintain, affording them time to rest and stay well. Neither of these conceptualisations of a garden is wrong, despite each person's conceptualisation being different to one another's. This is how I understand the experience of wellbeing in the lifeworld. Somehow, we are united in our understanding of what wellbeing means as a generic label, yet each of us holds a unique, person-centred idea of what perfect wellbeing entails for us.

This chapter has argued two things. Firstly, in much the same way that humans turn a house and garden into a home – distinct from the structured and monotonous design of show-home gardens – we bring our collective concept of wellbeing to life in a way that market conceptualisations, alone, cannot. Secondly, just as gardens rely on a mix of natural resources (like sunlight, rain, and pollinating lifeforms) and human interventions (like maintenance, green houses, propagation, and plant feed), our wellbeing is shaped by the make-up of our natural lifestyles and the targeted support of wellbeing services. Our role, as researchers and service-providers, is to develop our understanding of how to strike a balance between natural and targeted resources, and how we can support people to develop the garden (aka wellbeing system) of their own choosing.

This garden metaphor is something I wish for you to hold on to when applying the frames of communication discussed later in this book. The act of recording a communication framework in words makes that framework become static. But this is not what I want for you. I want you to approach Creative Health communication with a lens of intrigue and communication. For you to see my framework as emergent – a starting point for you to gain clarity from but also to build upon in your own work, to ensure it remains dynamic. This may become more readily necessary as your research or services develop over time, as your exposure to wellbeing lifeworlds will develop with each person you support. This knowledge is power. It is an invitation to treasure the fulness of those you support.

References

Angeler, D.G. and Allen, C.R. (2016) Quantifying resilience. *Journal of Applied Ecology*, 53(3), pp. 617–624.

Baynes, K. (2016) *Habermas*. 1st Edition. New York: Routledge.

Brown, T. and Katz, B. (2009) *Change by Design: How Design Thinking Transforms Organizations and Inspires Innovation*. 1st Edition. New York: Harper Business.

Deci, E.L. and Ryan, R.M. (1985) *Intrinsic Motivation and Self-Determination in Human Behavior*. Boston, MA: Springer US.

Gadamer, H.-G. (1975) Hermeneutics and social science. *Cultural Hermeneutics*, 2(4), pp. 307–316.

Galvin, K. and Todres, L. (2013) *Caring and Well-being: A Lifeworld Approach*. Oxon: Routledge.

Greco, M. and Stenner, P. (2013) Happiness and the art of life: Diagnosing the psychopolitics of wellbeing. *Health, Culture and Society*, 5(1), pp. 1–19.

Habermas, J. (1968) The idea of the theory of knowledge as social theory. In: *Knowledge & Human Interest*. Cambridge: Polity Press.

Hanlon, P. and Carlisle, S. (2016) The fifth wave of public health and the contributions of culture and the arts. In: Clift, S. and Camic, P.M. (eds.) *Oxford Textbook of Creative Arts, Health, and Wellbeing: International Perspectives on Practice, Policy, and Research*. Oxford Textbooks in Public Health. Oxford, United Kingdom: Oxford University Press, pp. 19–26.

Hayward, M. (2022) Level 1 training in narrative therapy. [In-Person Training] The Institute of Narrative Therapy. 3–7 October. Available at: https://www.theint.co.uk/training/level-one/

Holzman, L. (2014) *What's Critical Psychology? Look It Up!* [Online] Psychology Today. Available at: https://www.psychologytoday.com/gb/blog/conceptual-revolution/201403/what-s-critical-psychology-look-it [Accessed 12/05/2024].

Husserl, E. (1936) *The Crisis of European Sciences and Transcendental Phenomenology: An Introduction to Phenomenological Philosophy.* 6th pr. Evanston, Ill: Northwestern University Press.

Jackson, M. (2017) *How Lifeworlds Work: Emotionality, Sociality, and the Ambiguity of Being.* Chicago; London: The University of Chicago Press.

Kara, H. (2015) *Creative Research Methods in the Social Sciences: A Practical Guide.* Bristol: Policy Press.

Keane, N. (ed.) (2016) *The Blackwell Companion to Hermeneutics.* Chichester, West Sussex, UK: Wiley.

MacKinnon, D. and Derickson, K.D. (2013) From resilience to resourcefulness: A critique of resilience policy and activism. *Progress in Human Geography*, 37(2), pp. 253–270.

Martin, R.L. (2009) *The Design of Business: Why Design Thinking Is the Next Competitive Advantage.* Boston, Mass: Harvard Business Press.

Masten, A.S. (2014) Global perspectives on resilience in children and youth. *Child Development*, 85(1), pp. 6–20.

Morgan, D.L. (2014) Pragmatism as a paradigm for social research. *Qualitative Inquiry*, 20(8), pp. 1045–1053.

Quinlan, A.E. et al. (2016) Measuring and assessing resilience: Broadening understanding through multiple disciplinary perspectives Allen, C. (ed.). *Journal of Applied Ecology*, 53(3), pp. 677–687.

Schön, D.A. (1983) *The Reflective Practitioner: How Professionals Think in Action.* New York: Basic Books.

Toombs, S.K. (1987) The meaning of illness: A phenomenological approach to the patient-physician relationship. *Journal of Medicine and Philosophy*, 12(3), pp. 219–240.

Tschimmel, K. (2012) Design thinking as an effective toolkit of innovation. In: *ISPIM Conference Proceedings. The International Society for Professional Innovation Management.* Manchester: The International Society for Professional Innovation Management.

Ungar, M. (2018) Systemic resilience: Principles and processes for a science of change in contexts of adversity. *Ecology and Society*, 23(4), p. art34.

Williams, M. (2016) *Key Concepts in the Philosophy of Social Research.* Los Angeles: SAGE.

Chapter 7

Narrative Data

Creative Activities That Have Marketability Embedded in Their Design

Throughout my research into service-user engagement in healthcare, I have found there are a lot of data collection methods that account for service-users' voices, but an absence of studies which considers market restrictions in the way that data is collected. Moreover, whilst there are many research projects that invite service-users into the generation of data, rarely are they embedded into the data analysis process. With this in mind, I designed activities and collaboration guidance that can be used by researchers to improve their engagement with service-users.

These activities utilise oral true-life storytelling and directed questioning, coupled with visual prompting materials. The use of oral storytelling encourages spontaneous recollection of lived experiences, and the emotional recall associated with this style of storytelling inspires non-linear pattern-matching between memories. This pattern-matching provided me with insights into the aspects of participants' lifeworlds which shaped their perspectives and values, helping me to unravel new wellbeing links and context. Meanwhile, the visual prompts grounded stories in market-relevant frames, reduced my influence over how stories were told, and encouraged participants to code their own data. In this chapter, I will explain the theory and practice which prompted this development of activities.

Truth and the Lifeworld

My first consideration when designing data collection activities was the type of truth I was hoping to collect from the data. According to my lifeworld approach to wellbeing, different people hold different understandings of wellbeing and these separate understandings collate together to create a more refined and collaborative definition of wellbeing. Here, truthiness describes the quality of seeming or being felt to be true (Merriam Webster, 2025), which is the best way of describing the experience of each individual. Truth, on the other hand, might describe the concept of wellbeing once every person had contributed their truthiness. Since this model of truth relies on social negotiation, and because our social make-up is ever-changing, the truth I am striving

DOI: 10.4324/9781003423317-10

towards via my data collection activities aligns with the conceptualisation of Kara (2015). Here, truth is 'multiple, partial, context-dependent, and contingent' (p. 6). The best way to explore this truth is by 'looking intensely from multiple perspectives' (Sameshima and Vandermause, 2009, p. 277).

Practically, within a research project, we cannot interview every person that is alive, nor can we capture their changing views on wellbeing from one moment to the next. For this reason, 'truth' cannot be fully attained. However, there are design principles which will help to maximise the accuracy or meaningfulness of what we collect. For example, if truth relies on the compromise between diverse opinions, then data collection should aim to engage people from diverse backgrounds. This could involve socioeconomic background (which is a key determinant of health), ethnic background (which accounts for both cultural narratives and experiences of disparity), or other factors, depending on the goals of a study. Adding to this, activities can be designed to question how a participants' concept of wellbeing has changed over time and what contextual factors affected these changes. Both of these principles were applied to my recruitment and activity design.

In addition to information that can be collected via participant storytelling, concepts of wellbeing can be collected via health and academic literature. This once again diversifies the contributions of truthiness that define our shared understanding of wellbeing. By considering how participant stories align with – or disrupt – professional notions of wellbeing, throughout my data analysis, I was able to draw researchers and service-providers closer to the truthiness of society rather than the version of truth held within their discipline. Here, conflicts of opinion are not strictly signs of incorrectness, rather, they are expressions of unique experiences from people who can perceive only part of a greater picture at any given time.

A Fuzion of Horizons

With this version of truth in mind, the Creative Health Communication Framework can be considered co-constitutional (Koch, 1995), as the storytelling data that it is built from is a blended interpretation from the participants and myself rather than an infallible truth. This is labelled by Gadamer (1975) as a 'fusion of horizons' (p. 39).

Within a fusion of horizons, it is important to consider how power and positionality affect the collaborative nature of outputs. For example, Bakhtin proposes that the mind is a product of dialogical relations (Bakhtin, 1929; Bakhtin et al., 2011). If this is to be true, then who we are at any given time changes based on those we interact with and the social discourses these people refer to or rely on to make sense of the world (Hermans, 2001). In my work, I wanted to ensure that by own conceptualisation of wellbeing had limited influence on what participants prioritised in their storytelling. For this reason, I decided to incorporate visual tools – my logic being that it would provide a fairer basis upon which participant data-collection could be centred. Here, I could prompt participants to share more about their stories by referencing our shared activity intentions, rather than let my questioning be steered by the data I was most captivated by, or that which I resonated with or understood most thoroughly. Participants were also invited, at the beginning of our interview, to challenge the categorisations of these visual activities, should they conflict with their own nuanced conceptualisations of wellbeing.

However, even with these visual activities in place, my role in this reciprocal exchange is a complicated one. On the one hand, I limit my verbal involvement during the initial act of storying to avoid my own bias, beliefs, and values from overly swaying the content shared, yet by being a present observer I cannot remove my being from the act of storytelling. The order that information is shared, the moments that are emphasised, and the distance in which the participants hold themselves from their stories, are all affected by my presence in the room, my non-verbal reception of their information, and their perception of what information I find most important.

For this reason, I felt it important to shift the participants' perception of me away from researcher (and themselves as the researched) towards a more human and balanced exchange. To achieve this, wherever possible, I embedded community engagement into my recruitment strategy. This involved me attending community sessions, ahead of recruitment or data collection, so that the people who might be interested in taking part in the research project could first see me as a fellow community member. Moreover, by treating the data collection as a narrative development process – whereby each participant contributed their stories towards a collective narrative of wellbeing – the different types of knowledge between the participants and I were celebrated within a combined mission for change.

Collaborative Data Analysis

Wilson (2022) suggests that, in storytelling,

> an act of telling is simultaneously an act of listening (as one tells, one also actively listens) and an act of listening is an act of telling (in order to listen and create meaning, one needs to be simultaneously retelling the story).
> (p. 24)

In my position as a researcher, my role is primarily one of listening. If this also entails an act of retelling, then I wanted to ensure that I retold stories as accurately as possible. For this reason, I believe it is necessary to involve elements of Collaborative Data Analysis (CDA) in my work.

CDA is a term used by Jennings et al. (2018) to describe the act of service-users or target demographics getting involved in data analysis, evaluation, and design. This was identified as an area that was lacking in patient and public involvement (PPI) – a term used in medical spheres to describe consultation with service-users to help shape services and policy. The review found that whilst members of the public are increasingly engaged in the production of information, they are not meaningfully consulted in the reading of information. Two of the key limitations of designing for CDA is time and money – that is, people coming from non-research backgrounds will require new training, the work will need to fit around their other commitments, the project may need multiple people to analyse data at the same time making it a lengthier and discussion-heavy process, and lived experience expertise needs to be appropriately recompensed. However, in the absence of CDA, research is tainted by the assumptions and interpretive biases of the data analyst, particularly when it comes to storytelling data.

Responding to this, I developed a light-touch CDA approach. This involved designing data collection activities that incorporate the coding of data within the storytelling session. This means that individuals only code their own stories, rather than choosing thematic links across the dataset of participant interviews. This act of participant coding reduces researcher biases and offers the opportunity to seek clarifications during the interviews. For example, by referring to the coding structures within my clarification questions, I could reduce participants perception that I might be challenging their viewpoints, instead reassuring them that my questions were rooted in a desire to record the most accurate version of their perspectives. During the development of the Creative Health Communication Framework, the participant coding of their information allowed us to collaboratively unearth where nuances were held in their stories, to indicate where language structures may be of use in mental health promotions.

This act of collaboratively reassessing information to develop meaning aligns well with the pragmatist principle of 'iterative-cyclical problem-solving' (Stübing, 2012, pp. 590–591). When developing my own iterative methods of data collection and analysis, I referred to Morgan and Nica's (2020) Iterative Thematic Inquiry, whereby researchers recorded and developed thoughts using a reflective log. In my own version of iterative design, I chose to establish my thoughts in the creation of activity themes and headings, and then used these as a starting point for collecting more insights from my participants. A strength of this approach is that it acknowledges that preconceptions cannot be avoided. By prioritising the explicit recording of beliefs at the earliest possible stage of research, preconceptions can be interrogated throughout the process rather than being subconsciously incorporated during formal analysis. By developing activities that were informed by my understanding of market structures and their impact on wellbeing, participants could then challenge the legitimacy of these structures or comment on their alignment with their wellbeing conceptions. This ultimately led to more robust and considered design.

Activity One: The Importance of Contextualising a Lifeworld

Ahead of my two CDA activities, I wanted to start with an activity that gave context to participants' experiences of wellbeing – that is, their lifeworld. To achieve this goal, I drew upon a pre-existing exercise used within the field of Narrative Therapy. This exercise is called The Tree of Life, originally developed by Ncazelo Ncube and David Denborough (Denborough, 2008, pp. 17–98). It relies on a visual diagram of a tree, in which different sections stand for different elements of a person's character, values and lived experience:

Roots – identity labels, such as culture, favourite places, clubs they are associated with
Ground – regular activities they partake in, highlighting routines, hobbies, and mundane tasks
Trunk – the personal values and community values that shape their existence
Branches – their horizons, including hopes, dreams, and wishes (both for themselves and for those around them)
Leaves – people who are significant to them
Fruit – what legacies these people have left them
Flowers/Seeds – the legacies they wish to leave for others
[Optional extra] **Compost Heap** – powerful but negative forces can be placed here

By placing this activity first, participants did not need to keep readdressing the complexities of their context within each mental wellbeing story they told in activities two and three. This reduction in cognitive pressure provided them with the space to share what felt pertinent to them, with the trust that I already had some information as to why they might act or feel the way that they described. Another advantage to engaging with the Tree of Life activity, is that it provided a suitable degree of context to reduce my researcher bias, both within the facilitation of interviews and during the post-interview reading of data.

This decision aligns well with hermeneutic phenomenology whereby the reading of participant information moves beyond being purely descriptive to recognise the various cultural forces that shape experiences and their interpretation (Smith, 1987; Heidegger, Macquarrie and Robinson, 2007). It also accounts for the intersectionality of different individuals. Namely, as Esposito and Evans-Winters (2021) propose, 'qualitative inquiry from an intersectional perspective unashamedly and ardently concedes that individuals can be multiply situated in the world and, thus, the researcher must be prepared to accept complexity as a part of the research process' (pp. 1–24).

These sentiments mirror similar ideas that are carried within life narrative discourses. Raggatt (2006), for example, cautions that we should not assume a singularity of identity when people express life narratives. The Tree of Life activity is a great starting point for considering the complexity of human identify and experience, and how these shape an individual's conceptualisation of – and communication about – wellbeing.

Whilst this activity offered the least amount of codable data, it succeeded greatly in setting the tone of the interview to be calm, relaxed, creative, and trusting. One example of how interesting information was revealed, was through the identification of personal labels. Instead of seeing themselves in terms of traditional identity labels, such an ethnicity or gender, participants identified labels more important to them, such as 'truth seeker' or 'just like everybody else.'

Activity Two: Assigning Market-Relevant Metrics to Wellbeing Data

My second activity is the Scale of Influence (SOI). This is an eight-point numerical scale which asks participants to rate the degree to which different factors in their lives affect their wellbeing. This activity was an important tool for understanding the marketability of provisions as it showed which services participants genuinely needed and which factors they would rather deal with independently. This aligns to an important market consideration regarding 'satisficing.' Portigal (2013) describes 'satisficing' as a response to particular problems, whereby the pain of the problem is considered less annoying than the effort to solve it. In this scenario 'what [researchers or service-providers] observe as a need may actually be something your customer is perfectly tolerant of' (p. 5). This is an important consideration, as it highlights that the identification of a need is not the only ingredient for success. The financial cost of a service, and the emotional or time-related cost of engaging with it, are all necessary parts of strong market design.

Practically, the SOI activity worked by asking participants to describe their most positive and negative wellbeing stories out loud, with the intention of identifying contributing factors that they could write down on post-it notes/ or within digital note-boxes (depending on their method of delivery). These notes could be created whilst the story was being told or upon reflection on their story after it was shared, depending on the participants' preference. They had full control over what the factors were that they identified and how they were labelled. Once both stories had been shared, these notes were then distributed within the eight-column scale, whereby eight was considered most influential. Participants were encouraged to comment on the distribution of factors – in particular, where positive factors appeared in negative stories and vice versa. Dynamic reflections like these allowed the research to collect information that is particularly useful to service-providers.

One of the reasons that this activity focused on wellbeing at its best and worse was to make use of the psychology of change. Storr (2019) suggests that this type of differentiation can spark the interest of our narrative-led brains as it presents an opportunity to create a narrative about what changed and why (p. 11). In preparation for the participants interviews, I researched into narrative techniques such as *Unique Outcomes* (Matos et al., 2009) and *Moments of Coherence* (Parr, 2007) – each of which refer to a type of change within a dominant life narrative. By applying these theories of narrative, I could draw from participants natural enthusiasm for their dominant life-stories and harness it for the benefit of revealing enlightening information for the research.

Another benefit of discussing both best and worse wellbeing stories is that it encourages more truthful and vulnerable sharing of information from participants. Had I asked participants to describe their general wellbeing, they would likely have told a version of events that framed them in a good light, making themselves appear stronger or more attentive to their needs than they may be in reality. Whereas, in the model I chose, the difficulties they struggled with at their worst do not become the sole reflection of them, so potential stigma is diminished, whilst the successes they achieved at their best can be celebrated without skewing the reality of their experience. By describing two stories, it also provided space to account for evolving knowledge, self-reflection, and changing contexts.

A third benefit of this approach is that it can be analysed through both an essentialist and a constructivist lens, with consideration of scope and stability of wellbeing. If an essentialist model of wellbeing was the most accurate way of identifying areas of support, then I would expect the pool of participants to have fundamental needs that repeat throughout each of their SOI charts. By comparing their wellbeing at their best and their worst I would expect to see an absence of essential resources in the worst scenario and a presence of them within their best scenario. Comparatively, should participants' needs be heavily subjected to their values, socialisation, and environment, as expected through a social constructivist model of wellbeing, then I would expect to see disparity of needs, both in the factors identified and the scale of influence that they are attributed with. If a combination of these models were most applicable, I would expect to see some cross overs between participants from similar demographics or backgrounds but may observe deviation through the dataset at large. Since all these perspectives are permitted within this activity, it aligned with my attempt to remain epistemologically neutral wherever possible, to retrieve the most relevant data possible for a market-informed investigation.

Finally, a strength of this activity is that it provides a means for artistic service-providers to incorporate the logic of measurement into their design, whilst staying true to philosophies that celebrate subjectivity and meaning-making. Where their medical counterparts can more readily measure mental health based on their concepts of good and bad diagnosis, this subjective measurement approach prioritises the view of wellbeing held by the individuals experiencing it. What it measures, in the absence of a diagnosis, is the degree to which an individual believes their needs are being met and the access they have to supportive resources. This information is ultimately that which informs a service-user's market behaviour, making it highly compatible with a pragmatist study.

Activity Three: Compartmentalising Mental Wellbeing to Uncover Complexity

To complement these two activities, my final activity asked participants to re-organise the factors identified within the SOI activity into categories of wellbeing. The logic behind this is that the more that we can understand about these wellbeing factors, the more clarity researchers and service-providers can use in their communications.

Existing medical provisions market their value, both, by describing what they change and how they expect to change it (as demonstrated in the SSRI example provided in chapter three of this book). This allows for them to build trust with users, as their role becomes highly transparent and it is clear what the service-user can attain through the service-provider's support that they otherwise could not. Where medical practitioners can refer to biological markers for this, artistic providers typically offer changes that are conceptual, social, or incorporate elements of abstraction. My categories of wellbeing, therefore, offer a range of lenses through which they can discuss their services.

I chose to refer to these lenses as 'wellbeing orientations' – the logic being that, in the absence of resources filed under these headings, individuals can feel disorientated in a particular area of their lives. When we talk about wellbeing as one overarching experience, we can miss the subtleties of these wellbeing orientations and are therefore unable to design unique responses for each.

The seven wellbeing orientations I identified were:

1 Social
2 Environmental
3 Temporal
4 Physiological
5 Spiritual
6 Psychological
7 Ability to Orientate

These were built in response to a range of literature, three of which I will outline here as key examples. Firstly, there is Bulcock's (2019) *Five Factors to Building Resilience*, which are: Nourishment of the Body, Nourishment of the Mind, Nourishing Connection, Environments That Nourish, and Nourishing One's Time (pp. 93–160). Next are the *Five Ways to Wellbeing* which are promoted by the mental health charity *Mind* and the NHS. These are: connect (to get a sense of belonging), be active (to promote positive mood), take notice (to enjoy the world around you), learn a new skill (to boost confidence), and give to others (to provide a sense of purpose) (NHS, 2018, 2019; Mind, 2022). Finally, Galvin and Todres (2013) identify *Five Qualitative Dimensions of the Lifeworld*, which mirror these categories. These dimensions are: Temporality, Spatiality, Intersubjectivity, Embodiment, and Mood/Emotional Attunement (Galvin and Todres, 2013, pp. 26–30). In addition to these sources, I noticed themes of social wellbeing, biological wellbeing, spiritual wellbeing, and cognitive wellbeing emerging from my review of literature.

By asking interview participants to code their data into this table, I could achieve five important things. Firstly, in considering the placement of their post-it notes, participants were encouraged to think about their story from a different angle to the one in which they originally delivered it. This provided new insights and understandings, both for them and the project. Secondly, by asking participants to code their own data, unexpected categorisations could be discovered and discussed. This reduced any facilitator bias I might unconsciously hold, whilst strengthening shared understanding. Thirdly, my approach to participant co-creation allowed the table itself to be challenged, discussed and, if appropriate, re-designed, to reflect the orientations of participant's lifeworlds more accurately. Fourthly, by observing whether a factor made its way into one or multiple categories, the research was given an indication to the complexity of participants' wellbeing systems (explored more in the next chapter). This was also achieved, based on the spread of factors across the categories – whereby some participants held resources in every category and others experienced dominant categories of resources. Finally, by placing every participant's answers within the same table, they could be grouped – following the interviews – and compared to identify repeating needs. By challenging and developing the framework to better understand how factors carry distinctly unique meanings to different users, researchers and service-designers can better identify how their services meet the needs of diverse audiences rather than only those who share similar lifeworlds to their own.

Enriching the Participatory Experience

One final thing I wanted to discuss in this chapter, is how the act of participating in research can be enriched for those involved. One of the ways that I achieved this was by making physical participation packs for participants to explore and get intrigued by, ahead of the interviews. Participation packs were designed to set the tone by indicating the tea-and-biscuit style chat that I was trying to emulate within the interview. This was achieved through the inclusion of refreshments (tea, coffee, a biscuit, and a savoury snack). Additionally, the pack gave participants tangible materials to work with, inciting a sense of creativity that cannot be achieved through digital materials (Ponticorvo et al., 2020), helping them to develop an emotional connection to the project ahead of the interview (Nägele et al., 2020), and leaving them with a lasting resource/memory of their engagement (Culpin et al., 2021). This included three A3 diagrams which acted as points of reference during the activities, post-it notes, and pens. When these packs were tested with mock participants ahead of the main study, one of them shared that they made an audible 'ooo' as they opened the interview pack, adding that it provoked a sense of playfulness and excitement. Other positive feedback noted that the pack looked like the standard of the university rather than an individual researcher, which helped them to feel like they were part of something important and foster trust that the project had been well designed.

In addition to the participation packs, I researched into narrative learning to identify ways that I could offer reciprocal benefits for my participants. In connection to narrative learning, Goodson et al. (2010) propose:

> In a very real sense, the story constitutes the life and the self. Life and self are thus at the same time 'object' and 'outcome' of the story. What complicates the matter further is that the self is also the author of the story. All this means that the construction of the story – the storying of the life and the self – is a central 'element' of the learning process.
>
> (p. 2)

That is to say that by expressing stories and reflecting in the nuanced way that these activities were designed to provoke, participants are able to further their learning from their experiences, reflect on moments of joy and affirmation, and leave the interview with new ideas of how they would like to progress their life going forward.

Bruner (1990) argues that constructing stories is a practice that individuals engage in when they are attempting to make sense of their place in the world. He describes stories as things which are collaboratively constructed, in that our beliefs and values derive from socially enforced cultural expectations and perspectives, and thus are most meaningful when shared with others (Bruner, 1990). I deduce, therefore, that by being an active listener in the storytelling process and asking meaningful questions, researchers and service-providers can play an important role in collaboratively constructing or strengthening a participant's sense of purpose. By inviting participants to verbally share true life stories about wellbeing within this project – many of which may be stories they do not usually or ever share with others – they can learn about how their narrative retelling shifts around their expectations of the audience (in this case, a mental health researcher) and their perceived purpose of sharing.

To heighten my role as an active listener and collaborator, I partook in a counselling skills course ahead of the data collection stage of my research. This taught value constructs, such as Unconditional Positive Regard (Rogers, 1958; Raskin and Rogers, 2005; Jacobson and Blundell, 2016), and facilitation skills, such as probing questions, paraphrasing to seek clarification, and pausing to allow thinking time and expansion of commentary.

Spontaneous feedback, from almost all participants, demonstrated the positive impact these exercises had on the participants involved. Winnie (2022) stated, 'I must admit, I've said a lot more to you about my life than I've ever said to anybody before.' Samawah (2022) said, 'Thank you. This has been a really good opportunity. I've got… I think I have got to learn a lot about myself. It's like I'm looking at myself in the mirror.' Bodhi (2022) added, 'The whole experience was really liberating and enjoyable […] it feels like my mind's had a spring clean! Thanks, Jane, for your patience during the interview and helping me open up with my thoughts and feelings!' (Bodhi, personal correspondence). Moreover, Ekundayo (2021) shared that it meant a lot to them to finally be listened to, adding 'I appreciate you and everything you are doing.'

Conclusion

Within the introduction of this book, I advocated for the importance of service-user engagement within market design, saying that only the appraisers of value could truly capture the difference between service benefits and market value. I argued that where a service-provider can be engulfed by their enthusiasm for a service's benefit and made blind to its chances of succeeding within a marketplace, a service-user is aware of the intricacies of their needs which heighten or decrease the market value of this same service. The data-collection activities explored in this chapter were carefully designed to distinguish these differences within participants' stories. By engaging with coding exercises, participants were offered an opportunity to detail the intricacies of their needs in a way that service-providers might not appreciate otherwise. Accordingly, I regard participants as co-creators of the Creative Health Communication Framework, since their stories contributed to a collective imagining of wellbeing and informed what this framework considers important to human fulfilment.

References

Bakhtin, M. et al. (2011) *The Dialogic Imagination: Four Essays*. 18. Paperback Printing. Austin, Texas: University of Texas Press.

Bakhtin, M.M. (1929) *Problemy Tvorchestva Dostoevskogo*. Nordersted: Books on Demand.

Bodhi (2022) Interview with Jane Hearst.

Bruner, J. (1990) *Acts of Meaning*. Cambridge, MA, US: Harvard University Press.

Bulcock, D. (2019) *Have It All (Without Burning Out)*. Lancashire, UK.: authors & co.

Culpin, I. et al. (2021) Tangible co-production? Engaging and creating with fathers. *Area*, 53(1), pp. 30–37.

Denborough, D. (2008) *Collective Narrative Practice: Responding to Individuals, Groups, and Communities Who Have Experienced Trauma*. Adelaide: Dulwich Centre Publications.

Ekundayo (2021) Interview with Jane Hearst.

Esposito, J. and Evans-Winters, V.E. (2021) *Introduction to Intersectional Qualitative Research*. 1st Edition. Thousand Oaks: SAGE Publications, Inc.

Gadamer, H.-G. (1975) Hermeneutics and social science. *Cultural Hermeneutics*, 2(4), pp. 307–316.

Galvin, K. and Todres, L. (2013) *Caring and Well-being: A Lifeworld Approach*. Oxon: Routledge.

Goodson, I. et al. (eds.) (2010) *Narrative Learning*. New York: Routledge.

Heidegger, M., Macquarrie, J. and Robinson, E. (2007) *Being and Time*. Malden (Mass.): Blackwell Publ.

Hermans, H.J.M. (2001) The dialogical self: Toward a theory of personal and cultural positioning. *Culture & Psychology*, 7(3), pp. 243–281.

Jacobson, S. and Blundell, A. (2016) *Unconditional Positive Regard – What It Is and Why You Need It*. [Online] Harley Therapy. Available at: https://www.harleytherapy.co.uk/counselling/unconditional-positive-regard-what-it-is-and-why-you-need-it.htm [Accessed 15/05/2020].

Jennings, H. et al. (2018) Best practice framework for Patient and Public Involvement (PPI) in collaborative data analysis of qualitative mental health research: methodology development and refinement. *BMC Psychiatry*, 18(1), p. 213.

Kara, H. (2015) *Creative Research Methods in the Social Sciences: A Practical Guide*. Bristol: Policy Press.

Koch, T. (1995) Interpretive approaches in nursing research: The influence of Husserl and Heidegger. *Journal of Advanced Nursing*, 21(5), pp. 827–836.

Matos, M. et al. (2009) Innovative moments and change in narrative therapy. *Psychotherapy Research*, 19(1), pp. 68–80.

Merriam Webster (2025). Definition of truthiness. [online] www.merriam-webster.com Available at: https://www.merriam-webster.com/dictionary/truthiness

Mind (2022) *Five Ways to Wellbeing*. Available at: https://www.mind.org.uk/workplace/mental-health-at-work/taking-care-of-yourself/five-ways-to-wellbeing/ [Accessed 13/05/2022].

Morgan, D.L. and Nica, A. (2020) Iterative thematic inquiry: A new method for analyzing qualitative data. *International Journal of Qualitative Methods*, 19, p. 160940692095511.

Nägele, N. et al. (2020) "Touching" services: Tangible objects create an emotional connection to services even before their first use. *Business Research*, 13(2), pp. 741–766.

NHS (2018) *Mindfulness*. Available at: https://www.nhs.uk/mental-health/self-help/tips-and-support/mindfulness/ [Accessed 13/05/2022].

NHS (2019) *Five Steps to Mental Wellbeing.* Available at: https://www.nhs.uk/mental-health/self-help/guides-tools-and-activities/five-steps-to-mental-wellbeing/ [Accessed 13/05/2022].

Parr, H. (2007) Collaborative film-making as process, method and text in mental health research. *Cultural Geographies*, 14(1), pp. 114–138.

Ponticorvo, M. et al. (2020) On the edge between digital and physical: Materials to enhance creativity in children. An application to atypical development. *Frontiers in Psychology*, 11, p. 755.

Portigal, S. (2013) *Interviewing Users: How to Uncover Compelling Insights.* Brooklyn, New York: Rosenfeld Media.

Raggatt, P.T.F. (2006) Multiplicity and conflict in the dialogical self: A life-narrative approach. In: McAdams, D.P., Josselson, R. and Lieblich, A. (eds.) *Identity and Story: Creating Self in Narrative.* Washington: American Psychological Association.

Raskin, N.J. and Rogers, C.R. (2005) Person-centered therapy. In: Corsini, R.J. and Wedding, D. (eds.) *Current Psychotherapies.* Pacific Grove: Thomson Brooks/Cole Publishing Co., pp. 130–165.

Rogers, C. (1958) The characteristics of a helping relationship. *The Personnel and Guidance Journal*, 37, pp. 6–16.

Samawah (2022) Interview with Jane Hearst.

Sameshima, P. and Vandermause, R. (2009) Methamphetamine addiction and recovery: Poetic inquiry to feel. In: Prendergast, M., Leggo, C. and Sameshima, P. (eds.) *Poetic Inquiry: Vibrant Voices in the Social Sciences.* Berlin: BRILL, pp. 275–286.

Smith, D.E. (1987) *The Everyday World as Problematic: A Feminist Sociology.* 4. [print.]. Boston, Mass: Northeastern University Press.

Storr, W. (2019) *The Science of Storytelling.* London: William Collins.

Stübing, J. (2012) Research as pragmatic problem-solving: The pragmatist roots of empirically-grounded theorizing. In: Bryant, A. (ed.) *The SAGE Handbook of Grounded Theory.* Los Angeles: SAGE, pp. 580–602.

Wilson, M. (2022) *Storytelling.* First edition. Bingley, UK: Emerald Publishing.

Winnie (2022) Interview with Jane Hearst.

Chapter 8

Developing the Creative Health Communication Framework

Creative Health researchers and practitioners working in mental health and wellbeing want to do good via their services. But the ability to do good can be limited by poor communication and incomplete considerations about service design. The Creative Health Communication Framework supports those seeking to make a positive change, to do so in the most effective way possible via clear, explicit and diverse communication about compatible service design and delivery.

Fantastic research is already available, identifying the wide array of 'mechanisms of action' through which arts, culture, and leisure activities can positively impact health and wellbeing (Fancourt et al., 2021). This is a great resource for researchers and practitioners to describe the specificity of change they intend to catalyse, in a manner that health professionals will recognise and respect. Where the Creative Health Communication Framework adds to existing models for framing the benefits of Creative Health is in its prioritisation of how we communicate to members of the public. For this, it starts with broader categories than the mechanisms of action – i.e., categories that were designed to mimic the way that members of the public conceptualise and communicate their own wellbeing stories.

The Rationale for Developing a Creative Health Communication Framework

In the opening chapters of this book, I established the context that led to the development of The Creative Health Communication Framework. Here, I will summarise these arguments to present a clear rationale.

Firstly, there a rich and ever-expanding evidence base demonstrating how Creative Health services are able to positively impact priority health conditions and prevent other health issues. Despite this, there is not wide-spread recognition of them throughout society. This points to an issue relating to our market.

Our specific capitalist economy and healthcare culture/philosophy shape the degree to which Creative Health services can thrive in a marketplace

DOI: 10.4324/9781003423317-11

(Chapters 2 and 3). Moreover, service-users' enthusiasm and comprehension affect how much they will interact with services. I argue, therefore, that both the market system and service-users need to be satisfied for a Creative Health provision to thrive.

How we speak about Creative Health reflects and shapes the power dynamics in the sector (Chapter 4). Knowing this, we can begin to consider how communication might impact the degree to which the market system and service-users can feel satisfied with a Creative Health offering.

Looking at the market from a pragmatic viewpoint allows us to develop solutions that account for market forces in their design (Chapter 5). Accordingly, I looked for pragmatic ways that I could impact the communication that takes place within the wellbeing market, to encourage better representation of Creative Health activity.

I theorise that the communication of wellbeing within a marketplace is best described as 'market wellbeing' – a place of negotiation between the lifeworlds of individuals and the market system that they seek support from within (Chapter 6). From a pragmatic point of view, any solution would also be required to sit in this negotiation space, satisfying both the market system and service-users, and treating this as a dynamic and necessary relationship rather than two siloed entities of investigation.

Finally, my data collection procedure has demonstrated that there is a place for narrative in this pragmatic consideration. I question how we might unite the story of our market philosophy with the stories of individuals, through a common language.

This is where the case for a Creative Health Communication Framework is born. The more synergy we can create between the point of view of service-users, service-providers, and service-commissioners within our market system, the greater our chances of progressing Creative Health within the marketplace.

Positioning of the Creative Health Communication Framework

The Creative Health Communication Framework is primarily about improving promotional communication in relation to mental health and wellbeing services. By having researchers and service-providers consider this communication, there will hopefully be a secondary impact of improving service *design* of Creative Health activities too.

Promotional communication can mean different things to different people. In the introduction to this book, I defined it as 'any interaction between a researcher or service-provider and their service-users, participants, readers, or funders, whereby an opportunity exists to clarify their role and the strengths of Creative Health.' I explained that 'promotion is not, therefore, restricted to marketing material.'

The lens through which I have developed the Creative Health Communication Framework is designed around market wellbeing (as described in Chapter 6), which entails a trading of resources – either tangible or intangible. Accordingly, I consider Creative Health services to be **wellbeing resources.** However, I acknowledge that they are just one type of resource available – both in terms of their creative nature and because they are services rather than Creative Health activity that exists outside of the market.

For a Creative Health service – or any other wellbeing service – to be considered a valuable market entity, the resources offered through a service should be able to relieve a 'pain' that the service-user has, or produce a 'gain' they could not access in the absence of the service (Bland and Osterwalder, 2020). In the context of mental health and wellbeing, a **gain creator** might include greater fulfilment, a sense of purpose, visual stimulus, or emotional intelligence. A **pain reliever**, on the other hand, might include the reduction of loneliness, the reframing of harmful narratives, the alleviation of trauma responses, or improved rest patterns.

In the Creative Health Communication Framework, I conceive of **wellbeing** as the result of a well-functioning but everchanging wellbeing system (as described at the end of Chapter 6). This allows wellbeing to be considered within a market lens, as it asks the market what their role is in maintaining the function of that wellbeing system and whether the price of a service outweighs the cost that the system incurs in the absence of that service.

For this reason, I will frequently refer to **threats to wellbeing** throughout the Creative Health Communication Framework. These threats may describe something which is actively challenging the wellbeing of an individual or might point to the absence of a resource. This conceptualisation may not align with everybody's preference for how they talk about their wellbeing, so readers are invited to adapt the framework to their or their service-users preferences.

Finally, since I am concerned with Creative Health *services* specifically – namely anything which requires the exchange of money from either a commissioner/funder or service-user – I will predominantly use the terms **service-user** and **service-provider.** As outlined in the introduction to this book, Creative Health is not limited to services within a marketplace but the purpose of my framework is to support the compatibility and promotion of fundable provisions. As with the terminology of 'threats to wellbeing,' this conceptualisation may not align with everybody's preference for how they talk about their interaction with Creative Health provisions, so readers are invited to adapt the framework to their or their service-users preferences. Some common language used elsewhere includes, participants, artists, patients, individuals, lived experience experts, members, creators, and clients.

Development of the Framework via a Tiered System of Analysis

The framework was developed in collaboration with members of the public. Using the narrative exercises described in Chapter 7, I worked with them to explore their mental health stories and how they communicated about these experiences. Each person took part in a 2-hour semi-structured storytelling activity, using the Tree of Life, the Scale of Influence, and the Seven Orientations activities to prompt ideas and nuances. These activities took the same stories and asked the participants to view them through different lenses, inviting them to code their own storytelling data as they went along. What resulted from this was a breadth and depth of information, both from within the individual interviews and from across the cohort of participants. It was important to involve elements of participant-led coding in this exercise as it ensured that their stories were understood through their own preferred lenses. By recording data in this way, I not only had a range of language that I could compare to find a common language framework, but I could also check my own biases and assumptions about what these stories communicated and why. Once this check had taken place, I was then able to use my knowledge of the market to aid my identification of thematic areas of communication, evaluate existing language structures, and prioritise language frames based on their usefulness to both service-users and commissioners.

Throughout my framework development, I used a tiered approach to data analysis, 'looking intensely from multiple perspectives' (Sameshima and Vandermause, 2009, p. 227). This allowed me to contextualise participants' contributions within different epistemological perspectives and unveil which were most appropriate to identifying market insights. This comprehensive approach to design is described by Kostovich, McAdams and Moon (2010) as 'Universal Design' and Herriott (2014) as 'Inclusive Design' – both of which describe a process which 'open[s] up the broadest possible usability of a [design output] for very different users' (Wallisch and Paetzold, 2020). In my case, the design output in question was the Creative Health Communication Framework, which I wanted to be inclusive of as many people as possible and to align to market philosophies and practices as much as possible.

In the first analysis, I designed an approach entitled Narrative Compositional Analysis (NCA), which was made possible through the unique activity structures used within data collection. Here, I could interrogate whether any patterns emerged between participants' wellbeing charts, which could inform the creation of more specific categories of need. Whilst this generated interesting findings, the results demonstrated that participants' needs were unique and so did not conform to strict categories of language. The second analysis, therefore, analysed participant feedback and my observation notes from the research stage, to evaluate the suitability of the Seven Orientations (7O) language structure & Scale of Influence (SOI) parameters for use within the framework. The flexibility of these structured appeared to account for the uniqueness of participants' needs. To build on this, the third analysis drew upon knowledge from the literature to evaluate of the language of resilience theory. These evaluations were applied based on their applicability to participants' stories. Finally, I conducted a thematic analysis of the interview recordings, which accounted for any latent themes which had not been identified through the previous analyses but were relevant to a universally applicable language framework. Since I was looking for aspects of participants experiences which were commonly referred to in their narrative retellings, themes provided a useful means of recording these commonalities without necessitating a universally distinct relationship with them.

Key Findings from Each Analysis

My NCA functioned similar to scientific Compositional Analysis in that data was treated as relative information that forms part of a whole (Pawlowsky-Glahn and Egozcue, 2006). However, it differs from this traditional approach as the numerical indicators are subjective to the participants classification of their own data. Instead, I treated participants stories like work-in-progress pieces of art, which Golden (1986) expresses retain 'tangible residue of creation' which 'helps the viewer reconstruct the composing process' (p. 60). Here, elements such as balance, pattern, contrast, proportion, unity, and movement (Boddy-Evans, 2019) can be investigated to unveil information about the artist – in my case the participant storytellers and what they prioritise in their expression of wellbeing narratives.

I conducted two types of Narrative Compositional Analysis (NCA). The first combined all the data from the SOI and 7O activities into a table, whereby scale was indicated along the rows and orientation was indicated along the columns. Here, I looked for patterns across the cohort of participants. I also coded each person's individual 7O tables into positive, negative and interchangeable factors, to see if other patterns existed. I was looking for four possible patterns which might predict how people would likely feel:

1 the complexity of their life narratives
2 the range of wellbeing categories that were supported
3 the deviation between their most positive and negative experiences of wellbeing
4 the particular types of resources that appear within their tables

This first NCA identified that there were no clear patterns emerging between:

1 the type of resources identified within each scaled orientation box
2 the type of factors repeating through each orientation column
3 the type of factors repeating through each scale of influence row

This included:

a thematic content
b regularity/irregularity of the factor experienced
c number of positive and negative factors appearing

For this reason, there was no way of developing a universal list of protective factors or risk factors, as seen in studies focusing on resilience (e.g., Winter et al., 2012; Bonanno and Diminich, 2013). Instead, these findings indicate that experiences of wellbeing are unique to the individual.

The second NCA demonstrated a difference between complex wellbeing systems (those where factors appeared across multiple orientations) and simple wellbeing systems (where factors predominantly impacted one type of orientation). The analysis showed that within wellbeing systems that carried complex factors, the factors were often considered a transactional relationship with outside systems, whereby the mood of the individual can affect the resource and the resource can affect their mood. This compares to the systems which contained mainly simple wellbeing factors, where it was possible for external resources to impact only inwards and for internal resources to impact outwards through a process of re-orientation.

In the evaluation of the SOI and 7O for use in the Creative Health Communication Framework, I collated spontaneous participant feedback and my own observations from interviews to consider the main pros and cons for their use. The feedback was incredibly positive, with many participants saying that they shared more information to me than they would their own loved ones or support systems, and that this was largely down to the gentle facilitative power of these activities.

There were two changes that did develop from this evaluation. The first was the conversion of the seven orientations into an advanced model of wellbeing orientation, which has three tiers:

a the ability to orientate – which denotes the cognitive or social ability to use resources
b the remaining six orientations – which are obtained through resources that support survival
c six 'pleasures' – the same categories as the orientations, but with a focus on thriving and joy

This is explored more thoroughly in Chapter 11.

The second observation was on how the orientations were communicated. The academic version allows for a focus on orientation and disorientation, which makes clear how the activity conceptualises wellbeing, for the means of transparency, and how it aligns this conceptualisation to existing theories of resilience. However, when making this accessible to the general public, the language was altered to be more user-friendly. Namely, the language was altered to Social Influences, Environment, Time-Related Factors, The Physical Body, Meaning Making, and Mindset. This altering of language is an important part of research and service design, and emphasises the importance for my language framework to be used as a starting point of categorisation, not a copy-and-paste solution to language.

My evaluation of resilience theory intended to identify whether it was able to offer guidance on how to respond to the factors identified through the SOI and 7O frames. My primary criticism of resilience theory is that by encouraging market-users to aim for the ideal of resilience, the marketplace directs the conversation about wellbeing away from feelings of abundance, purpose, joy, and contentment, towards a mission to stay strong, productive, and accepting of infinite pressure.

When analysing participant data for occurrences of *resistance* I observed that there were fewer clear demonstrations within the interview data than you would expect to find if resilience – as it is currently theorised – was the most applicable way of understanding our wellbeing. Moreover, examples demonstrated a risk of:

1 diminishing the visibility of impediments to people that could help those in need
2 developing habits that put all external influences at arm's reach, restricting their access to positive influences
3 having a guard up during moments of safety, which prevented any negative forces that are contained internally from being released

My analysis of *resiliency* showed that the experience of wellbeing going up and down was not a bouncing motion that occurred once threats had been overcome, but a flowing motion that correlated to the persistent change in accessibility of resources. It also unveiled the importance of clarifying the co-occurrence of stability with high baselines of wellbeing. The implicit assumption in traditional resiliency is that stability is good and instability is bad. Participant interviews suggested this was an oversimplification. For this reason, I propose that reference to a Resiliency Measurement Matrix is more useful (Figure 8.1), as it demonstrates that a stable wellbeing with a low baseline should be considered to be just as disorientating as instable wellbeing with a higher baseline.

Adaptive capacity featured much more regularly in participants stories. My analysis demonstrated that adaptive capacity is dependent on a range of facilitative mechanisms. These include:

- an individual's self-awareness
- their ability to develop complexity within their moral concepts

- their access to tangible resources which can further their goals
- their appetite for self-development
- the degree to which their values conflict with normative or powerful value systems
- the frequency with which they apply long-term thinking
- their dedication to purposeful action
- their courage to allow things to get more difficult before they get better, or to engage with moments of discomfort
- problem solving skills and engagement with complex concepts
- facilitative environments
- access to memories or role models which demonstrate what can be

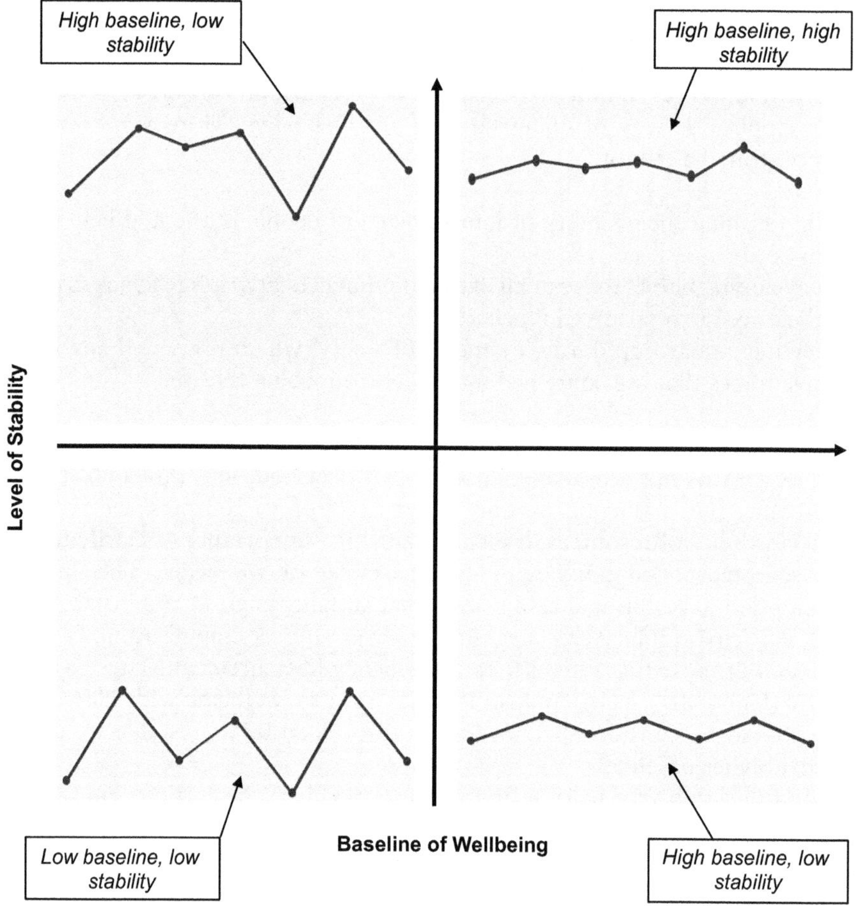

Figure 8.1 Resiliency Measurement Matrix.

- a willingness to experiment, be wrong, embrace chaos, and discover unexpected solutions
- the way in which the negotiation between self and others is prioritised
- time to develop learning

An individual did not need to hold all these mechanisms to engage with adaptive capacity, but the more mechanisms that they had access to, the more likely they were to be able to adapt.

In my analysis I also coined the term *adaptive choice* to recognise cases where enthusiasm is restricted by external barriers or where accessible change is not made use of due to personal choice.

Linked to MacKinnon and Derickson's (2013) criticisms of resilience theory, participants stories also show that internal resources, alone, were not enough. This led to the creation of a frame within my Creative Health Communication Framework which looks at internal and external resources. I could see how social discourses and values could negatively impact wellbeing, leading to another frame that looked at whether there was an absence of resources or a presence of misaligned resources. My analysis also led me to design the language of *internal abundance* and *internal deterioration*, which is explored more in Chapter 9.

My final analysis of participant data sought to unveil any important aspects of participants' experiences which were neglected in the other analyses. This was a thematic analysis, informed by Braun and Clarke (2006) design guidance. For this I looked for moments of surprise in the storytelling transcripts and activities. Examples include fascinating choices like Jiva categorising jail as a perfect environment, or Ekundayo choosing a moment of abuse as their example of greatest wellbeing. They include comments like that of Gayle who insisted that the context of the second world war provided some of their greatest happiness, and Kris's revelation that, should they pass them on the street, they would thank their abuser. These snapshots of life challenge the dominant narrative on wellbeing and, therefore, promised to offer new insights and opportunities to innovate the existing models of care used within the field. Once I identified moments like this from each interview, I filed them under a thematic title and the remaining interviews were then re-analysed to identify similar but less striking instances of this same theme. By combining lived experiences in this way, it offered me a rich description of these moments of deviation.

In total, I identified fifteen thematic groups through this analysis, six of which were turned into sections within the language framework, seven of which informed the framing of examples, and two of which identified gaps in the research which benefit from further consideration in future research projects.

Having completed all four of these analyses, I had a wealth of insights to draw upon within the creation of a language framework. These insights were grouped into three areas of inquiry – 1) **the threat to be addressed, 2) the solution to be deployed, and 3) storying the service offering** – and totalled 12 questions/frames (Figures 8.2 and 8.3).

The Creative Health Communication Framework	
Stage One: The Threat to Wellbeing	Internal or External Threats
	Scale of Impact
	Wellbeing Orientations
	Absent or Misaligned Resources
Stage Two: The Role of the Service-Provider	Identifying or Managing Threats
	Internal or External Resources
	Specific or Holistic Goals
	Resilience Strategies
Stage Three: Contextualising the Service	The Distinct Roles of Service-User and Service Provider
	Single Service or Collaborative Team
	Trust-Building and Attainability of Healthcare Services
	Promotional Voices: Scientific, Storytelling, or Poetic

Figure 8.2 Basic breakdown of the Creative Health Communication Framework.

Is the threat located internally or externally? *i.e., is the threat to wellbeing related to things like self-narratives and perceptions or issues with systems and environments*
How much does the threat impact wellbeing? *i.e., does the effort to endure the threat to wellbeing outweigh the cost of your service – whether that be financial, or relating to time and energy*
What type of disorientation does the threat create? *i.e., does the threat to wellbeing affect the individual's environment, social life, time, body, sense of meaning, sense of self, or is the threat disorientation in and of itself*
Is the threat caused by a loss/absence of resources or the presence of misaligned resources? *i.e., is the individual struggling because they cannot access the resources required to stay well, or are the resources they are accessing misaligned to their wants and desires*
Is the service provider's role to identify or manage threats to wellbeing? *i.e., are they helping service-users to unravel and understand what they are struggling with, or are they offering ways to mitigate these difficulties*
Does the service-provider's support help service-users to attain internal or external resources? *i.e., will the service be cultivating a stronger sense of self and a greater resilience, or can the service-provider access tangible resources or offer a particular form of advocacy that is difficult to access in the absence of the service*
Does the service-provider hold specific or holistic goals? *i.e., are they focusing on a precise aspect of wellbeing, or offering a more comprehensive package*
Is the service-provider informed by a particular resilience strategy? *i.e., are they helping their service-user to resist difficulties, bounce back from them, adapt in different circumstances, or identify existing resources that enable change*
Is there clear communication about the difference between the role of the service provider and the role of the service-user? *i.e., is the service-provider being treated like the trained expert, or is the service-user the expert by experience? And how does this shape the relationship?*
Will the service-provider be contributing to a set of collaborative support services or will they be supporting the service-user alone? *i.e., do you know the appropriate complimentary services to signpost to or collaborate with? Or will you be communicating the limitations to what you can offer alone?*
How does the service-provider plan to develop trust and make their service more attainable? *i.e., will you be responding to pre-existing stigmas about mental health and perceptions about healthcare? How will you re-establish trust with the disenfranchised?*
Can the service-provider identify the appropriate 'voice' to discuss tangible or intangible resources? *i.e., a scientific voice may be well suited to clinical audiences or when discussing tangible, measurable resources. A poetic or storytelling voice may be more appropriate when attracting service-users and appealing to emotive value.*

Figure 8.3 The 12 questions within the Creative Health Communication Framework.

Section One of the Framework: The Threat to Be Addressed

Here, the first question is: **is the threat located internally or externally?** Those using the framework have to option to design a research project or service which responds to:

1 an internal threat to wellbeing
2 an external threat to wellbeing
3 a combination of the two

The second question in this section is: **how much does the threat impact wellbeing?** Here, the framework can be applied in a numerical scale or a descriptive scale, i.e.:

1 the core problem to be solved
2 undue pressures which can be eased
3 background factors which do not impact significantly enough to require attention

The third question in this section is: **what type of disorientation does the threat create?** Answers to this question are tiered. Starting at the centre, researchers or service-providers may support those who, for some reason, lack to ability to orientate to the world around them. This might be due to physiological barriers such as brain injuries or degenerative diseases, or to systematic barriers such as demographics lacking the knowledge, language, or power to self-actualise. If the target research participant or service-user holds the ability to orientate, then the types of orientation they may wish to have supported include:

1 social
2 environmental
3 temporal
4 physiological
5 psychological
6 spiritual

These orientations are linked to the individual's survival and wellbeing. If they experience balance across these modes of survival, then creative activities may exist to help them thrive. This turns an orientation into a pleasure, and the six types of pleasures available mirror the six key orientations.

The final question in this section is: **is the threat caused by a loss/absence of resources or the presence of misaligned resources?** The potential answers in this section are:

1 recent loss of resources
2 ongoing absence of resources
3 misaligned resources
4 a mixture of the above

This can be ascertained through careful and inquisitive inquiry with research participants or service-users.

Section Two of the Framework: The Solution to be Deployed

Here, the first question asked is: **is the service-provider's role to identify or manage threats to wellbeing?** Here, the answer may be:

1 identify
2 manage
3 a mix of both

The second question in this section is: **does the service-provider's support help service-users to attain internal or external resources?** The possible answers being:

1 internal resources
2 external resources
3 both

The third question then goes on to ask: **does the service-provider hold specific or holistic goals?** The possible answers to this question include:

1 a single specific goal
2 a number of specific goals
3 holistic goals – that is, those that are non-descript, comprehensive but unable to be measured, or outcomes which change dependent on the person accessing support

If it is the latter answer, it is important for researchers and service-providers to describe their conceptualisation of holistic in the context of their work.

The fourth question in this section asks: **is the service-provider informed by a particular resilience strategy?** Here, answers may include:

1 resiliency
2 resistance
3 adaptation
4 development of functional diversity

5 nurture of internal abundance
6 resourcefulness
7 a mixture of multiple
8 a new approach to resilience

Section Three of the Framework: Contextualising the Service

In the final section of the Creative Health Communication, questions are asked to provide context to the service's offering. These are often pieces of information that researchers or service-providers assume are implicit, but for disenfranchised individuals, or those with access needs, extra thought is required in communicating these factors explicitly.

The first question is: **is there clear communication about the difference between the role of the service-provider and the role of the service-user?** The answers in this section are not an either-or, rather readers are advised to consider:

1 the role of the service-provider
2 the role of the service-user
3 the way that these boundaries are communicated and maintained
4 what happens in the scenario that these boundaries are crossed and how do you communicate these expectations in advance

Following this, the second question asks: **will the service-provider be contributing to a set of collaborative support services or will they be supporting the service-user alone?** Answers may include:

1 a specific function within a collaboration
2 multiple functions, delivered alone
3 a specific function, delivered alone

This question helps researchers and service-providers consider the safeguarding concerns that might arise and how these may be navigated or planned for.

The third question in this section is: **how does the service-provider plan to develop trust and make their service more attainable?** The question prompts support researchers and service-providers to consider a range of answers. These include:

1 being clear with the limits of a service
2 removing barriers to the service
3 indicating how the service differentiates from the limitations of others
4 reducing stigma of getting help

5 validating the service-users own experience and values through a person-centred approach
6 expressing boundaries within the helping relationship

Finally, the Creative Health Communication Framework asks: **can the service-provider identify the appropriate 'voice' to discuss tangible or intangible resources?** Potential answers to this question include:

1 scientific/ descriptive voice
2 narrative/ storytelling voice
3 poetic voice

Other voices may be available.

When using the Creative Health Communication Framework in your own work you will find that different questions/ frames will be more suitable to different research projects and services. It is not necessary to use every single frame in every communication you have, rather a strategic mix of frames can provide your participants/users or commissioners with a clearer view of what you offer. This clarity is something that may not exist in the absence of this information. The intention of the framework is to increase engagement with Creative Health services through better communication across the sector. It is hoped that this benefit will also be felt on the level of individual researchers and providers as you promote you own provisions.

Final Thoughts...

To conclude this chapter, I would like to quickly demonstrate how the framework removes some of the communication challenges that exist in its absence.

Let's imagine a theoretical service which uses dance to improve wellbeing. Wellbeing is a vast phenomenon, so service-providers might struggle to communicate how their dance provision is able to support a service-user through a wellbeing journey without knowing what they are struggling with in advance. I have heard practitioners complain about this need to know everything in advance, as it does not reflect the complex reality of their users, nor is it pragmatic to gather this information and respond within the commissioning restrictions of health providers. I argue that the answer is not to fight against the need for information, nor to give up on communicating. Instead, providers can focus on what they are able to communicate, which will offer commissioners and users greater clarity on what is on offer and, therefore, build trust in the service. Using the Creative Health Communication Framework as a guide, here are some examples from each section of what may be possible to communicate:

1 the topic will be related to an internal threat (Stage One: Question 1)
2 users will be supported via the identification of the user's internal resources (Stage Two: Questions 1 & 2)
3 the support will be offered through a lens of adaptive capacity (Stage Two: Question 4)
4 their role is in facilitation of the users own values (Stage Three: Question 1)

What is important about this is new mode of communication is that it shows that for provisions which lack a physiological indicator of change (such as heartrate tracking, cortisol decrease, etc) other important indicators are still available and should be prioritised in scenarios where they communicate more about the situation. To demonstrate, I will explore one final theoretical example.

Here the service is a narrative filmmaking therapy programme. The structure of this provision means that it takes place over a series of months, in a collaborative space, and it focuses on helping service-users to take control of their own stories. There is no obvious physiological indicators to measure the changes that are important to this provision, rather the change is expected to be in relation to life narratives and the way that they shape behavioural change.

Through the Creative Health Communication Framework, service-providers would be well equipped to describe:

1 that they are seeking to respond to social disorientation (Stage One: Question 3)
2 that this social disorientation has, in part, occurred due to a lack of social resources (Stage One: Question 4)
3 the degree to which this disorientation has been shown to impact their target demographic (Stage One: Question 2)
4 that they will be providing a form of holistic care (Stage Two: Question 3)
5 what makes this care holistic is that it addresses environment, time, and spiritual orientations as secondary impacts (Stage One: Question 3)
6 they will be working in a collaboration with talking therapists who will be responsible for the psychological orientation (Stage Three: Question 2)

Each of these frames provides clarity to users and funders without asking Creative Health providers to change the delivery of their service or their evaluation protocols.

As you can see in these examples, the Creative Health Communication Framework is able to capture the potential that is available within the arts and communicate this in a way that more closely speaks to artists' own passion and belief in their work compared to scientific means of promotion. You are invited to use it as a quick prompt, using the summarised view shown in this chapter. Or, for a more detailed understanding of how the framework can be applied, I invited you to read the latter chapters of this book – each of which explore a single frame.

References

Bland, D.J. and Osterwalder, A. (2020) *Testing Business Ideas*. Hoboken, New Jersey: John Wiley & Sons, Inc.

Boddy-Evans, M. (2019) *The 8 Elements of Composition in Art*. [Online] Thought Co. Available at: https://www.thoughtco.com/elements-of-composition-in-art-2577514 [Accessed 28/03/2022].

Bonanno, G.A. and Diminich, E.D. (2013) Annual research review: Positive adjustment to adversity – trajectories of minimal–impact resilience and emergent resilience. *Journal of Child Psychology and Psychiatry*, 54(4), pp. 378–401.

Braun, V. and Clarke, V. (2006) Using thematic analysis in psychology. *Qualitative Research in Psychology*, 3(2), pp. 77–101.

Fancourt, D. et al. (2021) How leisure activities affect health: A narrative review and multi-level theoretical framework of mechanisms of action. *The Lancet Psychiatry*, 8(4), pp. 329–339.

Golden, C. (1986) Composition: Writing and the Visual Arts. *Journal of Aesthetic Education*, 20(3), p. 59.

Herriott, R. (2014) Delimiting inclusive design. In: *International Design Conference 2014*. Dubrovnik, Croatia.

Kostovich, V., McAdams, D.A. and Moon, S.K. (2010) Representing User Activity and Product Function for Universal Design. In: *ASME 2009 International Design Engineering Technical Conferences and Computers and Information in Engineering Conference*. American Society of Mechanical Engineers Digital Collection, pp. 83–100.

MacKinnon, D. and Derickson, K.D. (2013) From resilience to resourcefulness: A critique of resilience policy and activism. *Progress in Human Geography*, 37(2), pp. 253–270.

Pawlowsky-Glahn, V. and Egozcue, J.J. (2006) Compositional data and their analysis: An introduction. *Geological Society, London, Special Publications*, 264(1), pp. 1–10.

Sameshima, P. and Vandermause, R. (2009) Methamphetamine addiction and recovery: Poetic inquiry to feel. In: Prendergast, M., Leggo, C. and Sameshima, P. (eds.) *Poetic Inquiry: Vibrant Voices in the Social Sciences*. Berlin: BRILL, pp. 275–286.

Wallisch, A. and Paetzold, K. (2020) Methodological foundations of user involvement research: A contribution to user-centred design theory. *Proceedings of the Design Society: DESIGN Conference*, 1, pp. 71–80.

Winter, Sue et al. (2012) *Visual Arts Practice for Resilience: A Guide for Working with Young People with Complex Needs*. Brighton: University of Brighton.

Part 3

The Creative Health Communication Framework

Stage 1

The Threat to Wellbeing

Chapter 9

Internal or External Threats

To develop a service/research project that has precise outcomes – that is, ones that are observable or measurable in some way – Creative Health advocates must begin by identifying what it is they intend to support. In the context of the Creative Health Communication Framework, this is achieved by exploring a 'threat to wellbeing,' via a series of four questions, until it is understood enough to be designed around. These questions move away from the pathologising of mental health experiences into labels and conditions, towards an exploration of a multifaceted state of wellbeing. This approach helps to clarify which part of an individual's complex experience they are seeking support with and better prepares professions to deliver an informed response. For service-users, it is this informed response which offers them added value against the provisions, lifestyles, or ideas that they can provide for themselves.

Is the Threat to Wellbeing Internal or External?

The first question in this exploration of wellbeing asks whether the 'threat' is internal or external. This question helps to describe the interaction an individual experiences between themselves and the world around them, and how this shapes the type of wellbeing that they experience.

External Threats refer to issues like poor housing or lack of access to green spaces, issues with physical health or even things like discrimination. These are factors that impact the *amount* of pressure that an individual endures day-to-day. The more external threats a person is faced with, the more they may experience a 'weathering' effect, whereby their physical health, mental health, disability-free years, and risk of mortality are negatively impacted by repeated exposure to adversity (Chen et al., 2023; Geronimus, 2023).

My understanding of external threats, based on interview data I collected from members of the public, is that they usually have a degree of universality to them in terms of whether people would be affected by them if

DOI: 10.4324/9781003423317-14

placed into that situation. A good example is that any person who is regularly exposed to mould in their home would be at increased risk of a respiratory disease (Baraniuk, 2023; Joffe, 2023; Wimalasena et al., 2021). As such, external threats are often coupled with an 'ideal' solution, which is informed by research into distinct outcome measures. Importantly, even in scenarios where this ideal solution cannot be achieved – either due to the limitations of the service-provider or the barriers that others put in their way – this sense of direction still proves useful in communicating value and generating movement in the direction of positive change.

Internal Threats, on the other hand, are shaped by an individual's values, perspectives, experiences, energy levels, and narrative interpretations. This is the type of threat that informs the *degree* to which an individual is affected by external threats. That is not to say that the individual is at fault in these scenarios, but that the complex layers of their experience have combined to create an instinctive preference for how they conceptualise and interact with the world around them.

Consequently, my understanding of internal threats is that they lack universality and, therefore, are in extra need of a person-centred response. This response is not able to rely on scientific evidence to the same degree as external threats; instead, research knowledge needs to be coupled with insights into an individual's lived experience. By addressing things such as internalised traumas, fears of being othered, or taught expectations of control and aspiration, individuals can slowly rewrite and overcome some of their automated responses to burden, in a manner that feels most meaningful and compatible to them. Only by making their care plan compatible with their sense of self can the impact of these services have an ongoing positive impact, that exists beyond the point of access to care.

One of the reasons why it is important to clarify whether a researcher or service-provider is prioritising an internal or external threat is that it affects their position when internal and external threats are in conflict with one another. To demonstrate, I turn to a story from one of my participants – referred to here as 'Devan.'

When Internal and External Threats Are in Conflict

Years ago, Devan experienced depression, following an accumulation of external threats including the death of one of their parents, their other parent getting Alzheimer's, the break-up of a long-term relationship, and an ill-fitting job.

Describing their experience of their depression, Devan said it was 'A kind of anger that's turned inwards' (Devan, 2021). This suggests that they also carried an internal threat. The sensation of this internal threat was clear:

'Everything's loud. [...] Every little thing – the banal everyday thing – was a big deal' (Devan, 2021).

As part of Devan's journey of healing, they released the tension of their depression in messy and inconvenient ways. They explained that the actions they needed to take to respond to the internalised aspect of their depression, negatively fuelled an external threat – that is, society's perception of them:

> I used to have this fear, if I went on a bus or train when I was in that mode, that this was shameful and humiliating. If I was going to start crying or start shaking, or whatever it was. And I've learned that you just do it; just let it be [...] letting things go is always better. The body needs to release things.
>
> (Devan, 2021)

Here Devan described a conflict between an action that was physiologically consistent with their mood, healing, and catharsis, but which is socially stigmatised. This demonstrates that at times there are not perfect ways to elicit good wellbeing; rather solutions are necessarily messy and in conflict with amalgamating a single thriving self. Devan demonstrates a clear position at the end of their statement, that they wanted to prioritise the externalisation of internal stress over the fitting into social expectations. For a researcher or service-provider to support somebody like Devan, they may benefit from mirroring this position. This would validate the journey that Devan has chosen for themselves and, therefore, reduce the external risk of ostracization via the creation of a trusted and supportive ally. This insight is particularly important for service-providers who may be working with disadvantaged demographics, as this permission to put the inner self before societal roles may conflict with the messages that individuals have received until then.

Distinguishing Clear or Complex Wrongdoing

For researchers or service-providers who might be unclear about the extent to which their role should respond to internal and/or external threats, it may be useful to assess the type of wrongdoing that is being experienced by an individual they are seeking to support.

Clear wrongdoing describes a negative action which exists outside of an individual, where there is a distinct boundary between what the individual stands for and how this action fails to meet those standards. Whilst these threats can be substantial in their form, the clarity of the wrongdoing makes them easier to process and endure.

Complex wrongdoing, on the other hand, can either describe actions that an individual feels at least partly responsible for, or a part of the individual's personhood which they deem to be a problem. Because these wrongdoings affect the individual on a more personal level, they are more difficult to rationalise or escape from.

I created these categories in response to some of the more surprising stories shared by participants. Here, storytellers spoke of moments where their environment was very bad, yet their wellbeing was notably high. For example, during Gayle's reflection on their experience of WW2, they shared, 'It was really the happiest time of my life although there was war on' (Gayle, 2021). The more that I explored these types of stories with participants, the more I noticed a pattern between those who experienced clear wrongdoing, matched with higher wellbeing, and those that experienced complex wrongdoing, matched with lower wellbeing. Within stories like Gayle's, which could be considered clear wrongdoing, participants demonstrated their ability to compartmentalise and endure contexts which were explicitly bad. The wrongdoing – in this case war – was clear, and there were other aspects of their lives that the individuals were more connected to, which provided them a sense of joy or purpose. This compared to other stories where issues of the external world were internalised; where the wrongdoing became more complex and, therefore, erosive.

By revisiting some of the participants' stories about more complex wrongdoing, I invite you to consider the importance of the person-centred approach to mental health and wellbeing; accepting individuals for who they are and how they interpret their unique experiences, so that we are better able to respond to them in a meaningful and validating ways.

Complex Wrongdoing in Experiences of Racism

Throughout Devan's life they have experienced a large amount of racism. This racism had a 'profound effect' on how they viewed themselves growing up (Devan, 2021). Recalling their earlier experiences, Devan labelled themselves as a 'conflicted teenager' and explained 'When things went wrong, it was my fault. And [I would think] it's because I'm black... it's because I'm this...' (Devan, 2021). Detailing the way that this racism was internalised, Devan added:

> Being brought up seeing yourself represented negatively in all media. And as a caricature or gross, you know, it was 70s [...] You start to think, well, as a black person what did we ever do [...] because we're not taught all this.
> (Devan, 2021)

To foster a better relationship with themselves and improve their wellbeing, Devan needed to access a resource which could re-externalise the racism. Luckily for Devan, during their experience of further education, they learnt about sociological theories. These provided Devan with a new perspective and this led to the re-externalisation of racism and the re-conceptualisation of it as a clear wrongdoing. Devan emphasised just how important this type of resource is for people who experience discrimination for being black, female, gay, or working class:

> If I didn't get engaged with feminism, if I didn't get engaged with socialism and union activity, and didn't [...] learn about sociology, and you know, public policies and how they affect people, I'd be that person; still going around thinking things are my fault, 'Everything's my fault,' 'I'm a bad person', or 'I've had the misfortune to be born [who I am]'.
>
> (Devan, 2021)

As you can see through this example, complex wrongdoings can turn an external threat into an internal threat, making it more difficult to respond to and flourish. This is particularly evident if we compare Devan's example to Bodhi who has experienced racism without it having an impact on their wellbeing.

At a school age Bodhi was spat at and bullied. They explained that they accepted this racism because it was happening everywhere at the time (England, in the 1970's). Bodhi clarified that one of the reasons why these racist acts were not internalised is because they had such a clear memory of their earlier childhood in Zambia, where there was a strong lack of discrimination. This acceptance of difference – including caste, religion, and otherwise – allowed Bodhi to view themself as equal, and the racist actions as matters of opinion from people they did not know or care about (Bodhi, 2022).

We can see through this comparison that the negative consequences of a threat like racism depend, somewhat, on a person's perception of discrimination and how much these messages are internalised. It is important to note, however, that internalisation of racism is not the only factor that shapes its effect on the individual. In Devan's story they gave examples of when discrimination had prevented them from accessing the same resources as others around them (Devan, 2021). Bodhi, on the other hand, expressed that the racism they experienced had little impact on their ability to self-actualise (Bodhi, 2022). This is why it is important for a researcher or service-provider to be clear on what aspect of a threat (i.e., the internal or external aspects) they are hoping to support, and how this shapes the complexity of wrongdoing experienced by an individual they are supporting.

Distinguishing Internal Deterioration from Internal Abundance

Importantly, the conversation of internal and external threats is inherently relational. For some, it is useful to consider the ways that our external experiences shape our internal wellbeing. For others, however, this outward-in conceptualisation of mental health and wellbeing was one that did not resonate. These were people who were less likely to engage in a study about mental health and wellbeing as they preferred to view their joy as self-made rather than socially determined.

To pay recognition to the type of positionality that these individuals preferred, I invite you to consider two final key terms: internal deterioration and internal abundance.

Internal deterioration is the result of embodied pressure. This internalisation can be the consequence of unrelenting external burdens, which distort and depreciate an individual's sense of purpose, joy, or direction. Alternatively, it may result from a weak or negative sense of self, which is easily impacted by the whims of the external world. Here, threats impact far beyond the immediate emotional level, into a person's ongoing wellbeing. Once this wellbeing is affected, everyday activities become harder to face and exceptional struggles corroborate a pre-existing narrative of suffering.

Internal abundance describes a wellbeing system which contains self-cultivated joy and a self-led sense of identity. This means that when external pressures impact an individual, they are still able to maintain hope, ambition, and optimism. This is because these resources of joy and strength are distinct from external burdens or opinions of their worth, which provides the individual with a higher and more resilient baseline of wellbeing. Within a state of internal abundance, individuals can recognise the rich world that lives within them that is separate to the material world. Whilst this does not make them immune to the burdens of the external world, these burdens are more likely to impact them at an emotional level rather than disorientate their long-lasting mood.

Crucially, these terms are not intended to reflect permanent states of being, and a person should not be considered inherently responsible for when they are able to harness internal abundance or when they are struck by internal deterioration. However, the terms do describe a prolonged period of perception which is shaped by an individual's relationship to the threats they encounter.

In some cases, it is possible for an individual to strive towards internal abundance. By recognising this headspace as a target destination, individuals can be inspired to act in ways which cultivate a wellness-producing lifestyle. Consequently, internal abundance can be a powerful lens through which researchers and service-providers can connect with the individuals they are supporting, to consider what an abundant life may look like for them and what resources – both tangible and intangible – are needed to create that life.

To illustrate the place of internal deterioration and internal abundance, within an experience of internal and external threats, I turn to two final examples from participants in my research.

Internal Deterioration/Abundance in Experiences of Abuse

When Ekundayo lived with their emotionally abusive parent, they described themselves as 'feeling insane' (Ekundayo, 2021). They explained that the abuse involved so many mind games that Ekundayo struggled to understand the extent of the wrongdoing and their identity within it. The most damaging part of this experience was the internalisation of the abuse which led to internal deterioration.

In comparison, Ekundayo struggled less with the abuse after their first child was born. This was because their child gave them a strong sense of purpose, and raising their child allowed Ekundayo to demonstrate what good parenting looked like to them (Ekundayo, 2021). At this time, the abuse from their parent continued, alongside abuse from a partner and issues with homelessness. Despite this, Ekundayo described this time as one of their happiest. This was because the revelations associated with their new-born child marked a significant shift in how they viewed their identity and sense of future (Ekundayo, 2021). In other words, they had reconceptualised their parent's abuse as clear wrongdoing and could, therefore, externalise a great portion of the trauma. This made it an external threat, which helped it to alleviate some of its imprint on Ekundayo's daily experience.

Another story of abuse came from Kris – this time, of a sexual nature from one of their parents.

'I'm gonna sound nuts' said Kris, 'but I've said it time and time again; if I could turn back time, I would let it happen all over again. Because it's been so pivotal in my life' (Kris, 2021). Describing the way that their trauma shaped their ability to empathise, meet the needs of others, and rapidly adapt, Kris explained:

> When people say, [...] 'I don't know where it'd be if this great thing hadn't happened'. [Well,] *I* don't know where I'd be if *that* hadn't happened, because my life has transformed in such a positive way ever since. [...] The amount of intelligence that it took at a young age to keep that a secret and to manoeuvre through life, without anyone knowing [...] And to still perform at school to a level that no one's going to worry about [...] go through puberty and all these confusing stages of life and not break, right. Like, that all came from having to deal with that.
>
> (Kris, 2021)

Kris explained that part of the reason why they were able to take positives from their awful experience was because they conceptualised their abuse as a problem with their abusive parent, rather than a reflection on their own worth (Kris, 2021). Throughout their story Kris focused on what they *could* control from their live, in an effort to develop their internal abundance.

This distinctive story, candidly expressed by Kris, further corroborates the notion that individuals who are responding to clearer wrongdoing may be better able to compartmentalise the threat and thrive, despite its existence in their life. However, it is important to note that the external nature of Kris's experience *did* improve once their abusive parent was jailed for their actions and removed from Kris's life (Kris, 2021). Moreover, an individual's response to a clear wrongdoing does not negate the wrongness of these actions. But by treating the abuse as a clear, external threat, Kris was able to protect themselves from the internalisation and despair that might have otherwise affected their ability to achieve self-actualisation.

Fascinatingly, Kris went as far as to suggest that, where others experience Post Traumatic Stress Disorder (PTSD), they have been lucky enough to experience Post Traumatic Growth (PTG) (Kris, 2021). This is a term that also comes up in academic literature in the field of psychology. Richard Tedeschi, one of the co-creators of the term, explains that 'People develop new understandings of themselves, the world they live in, how to relate to other people, the kind of future they might have and a better understanding of how to live life' (Collier, 2016). In Kris's case, their PTG meant that they had a heightened awareness of their behaviours and others' interpretation of them within a social setting. Kris was able to hold a complex awareness of how they were feeling and control these emotions based on how they wanted to develop their narrative or shape others' perceptions of them. These skills have continued to support Kris, long after their abuse, allowing them to apply them to contexts that are healing, self-actualising, and inspiring to others (Kris, 2021).

Applying the Learning to Creative Health

To demonstrate how this consideration between internal and external threats can be applied to Creative Health provisions, I close this chapter with two examples of Creative Health in practice.

The first example I share with you is in relation to banner-making. Artists such as Alaa Alsaraji, Jane Thakoordin, Jennifer Reid, Sabba Khan, and the Protest Props Collective build crafts in imaginative ways with the purpose of advocating for social justice and dismantling oppressive structures. One of the ways this is achieved is via banner-making workshops, where participants can create for protests and/or everyday signage. The focus of this work is inherently *external* as it focuses on strengthening collective values and challenging social injustices. Banner-making encourages reflection on what matters, what participants want to fight for, how they best communicate that, and it allows participants to collectively bond via crafts. The conversations shared during this crafting time provide practical and emotional support in relation to protesting, message development, and safety. The impact that banner-making workshops has is a reduction in feelings of powerlessness, better coordination of collective advocacy, and the long-term impact of social change, which provides for a better emotional landscape for those affected by social injustices.

The second example I share with you is in relation to somatic movement. Somatic practitioners include Oluwaseun Olayiwola, Poonam Dhuffer, Tania Nishi, Gemma Lucas, Rosie perks, Char Bailey, and Emma Money-Kyrle. This practice involves moving the body and/or making targeted sounds to reduce pent up stress and emotions and to improve *internal* self-awareness. Somatic movement classes show participants how we typically bias our thoughts over our feelings, and how this can cause trauma to build up in the body. These classes provide a safe space to release this bodily tension. They provide a collective sense of self-empowerment and a sharing space for healing journeys, without having to share what each individual is feeling or healing from. The impact of somatic movement is that it reduces somatic tension and supports the holistic processing of traumas. It reduces stress which leads to less fogginess of mind and lower risk of physical health complications such as heart issues.

As you can see from these two examples, the act of distinguishing between provisions that support internal or external threats to wellbeing provides a clear image of how they differentiate from one another. For people who may be struggling with issues like racism or abuse, as explored elsewhere in this chapter, both of these services have something to offer. This is one of the reasons why I believe that these frames of communication are particularly important. This clarity in what each service offers, allows a service-user to see that these services are not in competition to one another but rather supplement each other in a holistic package. This increased awareness of what creative health provisions can provide, supports service-users in making informed decisions about which services they engage with and helps them to understand their own threats to wellbeing in a more nuanced manner.

For readers who wish to apply this frame to their own work, you may find it beneficial to follow a similar format to what I have done in these two creative health examples. First, I started by introducing the provision. I chose to do this by outlining some prominent practitioners who work in these art forms. You might choose to add details such as where the provision is based or some of the topics that have been explored previously, or how it is delivered in terms of in-person or online. Secondly, I gave some context to the provision by linking it to an internal or external threat. You can choose to be specific or indicative here, based on what is most appropriate to your own provision. Thirdly, I gave a description of how this Creative Health intervention addresses the threat to wellbeing. I followed this by explaining the impact this has in both the short and long terms.

This structure may resonate with what you are trying to communicate, or the topic of internal and external threats may, itself, inspire an innovative approach of your own. Either way, the clarity that is offered through this distinction helps your promotional material and service design to be improved, in quality and clarity, making your work more commissionable and attractive to users.

References

Baraniuk, C. (2023) The doctor forcing landlords to act on mouldy homes. *BMJ*, p. 698. https://doi.org/10.1136/bmj.p698

Bodhi. (2022) Interview with Jane Hearst.

Chen, J.C., Pawlik, T.M. and Obeng-Gyasi, S. (2023) Internalizing social determinants of health: The ecosocial and weathering theories. In: Obeng-Gyasi, Samiliaand Pawlik, Timothy M. (eds.) *Social Determinants of Health in Surgery: A Primer for the Practicing Surgeon*. Amsterdam: Elsevier.

Collier, L. (2016) Growth after trauma. *Monitor on Psychology*, 47(10). https://www.apa.org/monitor/2016/11/growth-trauma

Devan. (2021) Interview with Jane Hearst.

Ekundayo. (2021) Interview with Jane Hearst.

Gayle. (2021) Interview with Jane Hearst.

Geronimus, A.T. (2023) *Weathering: The Extraordinary Stress of Ordinary Life in an Unjust Society*. London: Little, Brown Spark.

Joffe, T. (2023) Safer housing for better health. *BMJ*, p.597. https://doi.org/10.1136/bmj.p597

Kris. (2021) Interview with Jane Hearst.

Wimalasena, N.N., Chang-Richards, A., Wang, K.I.-K. and Dirks, K.N. (2021) Housing risk factors associated with respiratory disease: A systematic review. *International Journal of Environmental Research and Public Health*, 18(6), p. 2815. https://doi.org/10.3390/ijerph18062815

Chapter 10

Scale of Impact

During my consultation with members of the public, I used an activity called 'Scale of Influence' (discussed previously, in Chapter 7). Participants who engaged with this activity commented that they benefitted from the way that the scale breaks down their complex experience of wellbeing into manageable, co-occurring influencers and the degree in which they each impact their wellbeing. For this reason, I have also included the language of scale into the Creative Health Communication Framework, focusing here on *Impact*. What I will discuss in this chapter is how you can convert the numerical version of the scale into promotional communication. This will help you and your collaborators to paint a transparent picture of what you can support and to what degree, allowing your service-users to compare this against their own needs and their weighted importance.

Converting the Scale of Influence into the Scale of Impact

When promoting a service to commissioners or service-users there can be a mismatch between how you understand your service to impact participants and how much others expect your service to benefit them. Using scale in your promotional communication demonstrates self-awareness of where your service's strengths and weaknesses lie, it provides the person you are communicating to with points of reference, and it acknowledges how the degree of benefit is shaped by different budgets and context. The Scale of Impact can, therefore, be used as a tool for negotiation and business planning, a tool for exploration and health literacy, or a tool for transparent promotion. In the first case, the Scale of Impact provides a tiered approach to delivery, depending on how much budget is available to fund this delivery. By showing the increased benefit available, you may be able to demonstrate that greater investment also equals a greater return on investment – that is, that for every £1 invested, there is a monetary or social return larger than £1. In the case of exploration and health literacy, you can use the Scale of Impact to help those you support to better understand their coexisting needs, help them to plan ahead for moments of increased strain, and reduce the stigma associated

DOI: 10.4324/9781003423317-15

with their wellbeing. Finally, in the case of promotional communication the Scale of Impact supports researchers and service-providers in identifying their place within a market full of provisions. Research outputs and service offerings become comparable to other Creative Health, medical, or community offers and the distinguishing features can be celebrated.

Fundamental to this consideration is the understanding that wellbeing systems are dynamic relationships between different types of threats. Consequently, their impact on an individual's wellbeing is interrelated. By recognising that different threats cause different degrees of impact on this system, researchers and service-providers become more able to understand the issue/s they hope to solve or alleviate. This will help you to manage the expectations of your service-users and develop a more meaningful relationship as a consequence.

The Scale of Impact as a Numerical Scale

The degree of impact that a provision provides can be indicated in numerous ways, depending on the context of its use. When working one-on-one with a service-user, numerical scales can be useful tools in communicating how much a particular threat is impacting a user's wellbeing and how much this compares to other threats they are experiencing. This allows service-providers to align their subjective impressions of wellbeing to their users', prioritise what and when things are offered in a support package, and manage resources effectively.

The act of encouraging individuals to predict and problem-solve around their wellbeing can be very empowering, as it helps them to focus on the state of their resources and what they can do, rather than be passive observers of their story or fixated on what they can't do. This can also be used to elicit empathy for others who carry greater or alien burdens to them, thereby reducing the stigma associated with other people's wellbeing.

Another benefit of applying this numerical scale is within the context of an individual's story across different moments of time. Here, the same and different threats can be compared over time and understood better, thereby painting a more realistic picture of the person's ability to withstand difficult times, recover, or adapt.

Ultimately, in both of these scenarios, the Scale of Impact is used as a tool to better understand the parameters of a story or situation and the information that falls within these parameters. To illustrate, I provide two examples from participants.

The Use of a Numerical Scale to Reduce Stigma

In a discussion about wellbeing, one of my research participants, Samawah, outlined the different factors that were negatively affecting their wellbeing. They indicated the degree of influence that each factor had on their wellbeing using an eight-point scale. Here, eight indicated a highly influential factor.

Through this activity, Samawah was able to observe that they had a lot of negative factors scored in the 'highly influential' side of the scale which helped them to visualise the extent to which their co-existing burdens were affecting them. By engaging with the activity in this way Samawah became more accepting of the reasons why they were struggling. Their narrative stopped being one of weakness and moved towards an awareness that the pressures they were currently carrying were more arduous than those experienced by others around them (Samawah, 2022).

Similarly, when exploring a moment of higher wellbeing and the resources that provided them with strength, Samawah commented 'I have not yet found the number eight, so I'll just keep that blank I guess' (Samawah, 2022). This reinforced their new, alternative wellbeing narrative, as their difficulty with feeling strong was not a result of their worth but of their lack of access to strengthening resources.

The Use of a Numerical Scale to Plan Ahead

Using the same eight-point scale, another research participant, Aje, was able to identify which resources they were dependent on to manage the restrictions of their disability and prevent the erosion of their wellbeing.

Having identified a large number of complex factors, many of which were high scoring, Aje was able to consider how they might manage their wellbeing if any of these resources were removed. Whilst daunting at first, this consideration gave Aje insight about the type of routines and resources which provided them with the most joy and support. By improving their health literacy in this way, the Scale of Influence helped Aje to pre-emptively strengthen areas lacking in resources (Aje, 2022).

These are just two examples of unplanned benefits that resulted from using the Scale of Influence activity to heighten participants' mental health literacy. By using tools like these within communications, researchers and service-providers can be better equipped to understand the complex needs of those they support. Additionally, service-users and research participants can become more aware of the strengths and limitations of the support systems they access and, together, the interaction can achieve its utmost potential.

The Scale of Impact as Descriptive Language

Designating Scale of Impact is also useful within marketing promotions as it helps a service-user understand the type of wellbeing support they are likely to receive. In this context, numbers are less useful, as the audiences accessing this marketing material will each have different notions of what the numbers indicate. Moreover, using numbers to indicate Scale of Impact within an advertisement may give the wrong impression that these numbers describe the quality of a service. In this case, scale can be suggested by using indicative language.

For example, one service might seek to 'solve' the 'root cause' of poor wellbeing whilst another service may, instead, promote their ability to 'alleviate pressure' or 'provide spiritual replenishment.' In the first scenario the service-provider indicates that 1) they will be focusing on the most prominent and impactful need, 2) they are taking a great deal of responsibility within the individual's journey, and 3) the user can expect to see a large change throughout the process, along with a definitive end to their problem. The second scenario, on the other hand, draws attention to their ability to 'empower' the user and make them able to feel more ready to solve their larger issues alone. By indicating what level of wellbeing a service supports, service-providers are more likely to attract users that align best with their offering. This will improve the rate of satisfaction achieved by their client base, which will, in turn, support word-of-mouth promotions and high-ranking reviews online.

Using language like this to indicate a service-provider's role carries numerous benefits for the Creative Health sector at large. For example, if service-users are deciding between two interventions, they may choose one at the expense of another if they are both promoted as affecting wellbeing in a generalised way. However, if one service emphasises making a person feel stronger and the other focuses on solving a problem that requires this strength, their interdependence becomes clearer, encouraging the user to engage in both.

Another benefit of this language is that it improves the health literacy of the general population. By appreciating that multiple, co-existing issues may impact their wellbeing, and how these issues are affected by different services, members of the public can be more mindful about what it is they are trying to solve and what is the best means for them to solve it. These solutions may be innovative solutions they can create for themselves, making their wellbeing more sustainable, or the solutions may come from new unexpected providers, such as Creative Health practitioners. In the latter scenario, service-users are provided with the language to understand the value of the arts in healthcare and can make a comparison to existing services which have not worked for them in the past.

A final benefit that I want to highlight is the place of this descriptive language within leveraging conversations with commissioners. This becomes particularly useful for service-providers who are capable of offering a range of services, dependent on the resources provided to them. To illustrate what this descriptive language might look like in practice, I have provided two more examples.

The Use of a Descriptive Scale within Tiered Commissioning

To better understand the practical application of the descriptive language within tiered commissioning, I will be exploring three levels of artistic intervention that can be used within hospitals. The examples are inspired and informed by real examples that are delivered across the National Arts in Hospitals Network (NAHN). My comparison will demonstrate how varying levels of investment can impact the feasibility and outcomes of complex provisions, whilst also highlighting the value of low-cost options when resources are limited.

Lower Impact – Hospitals are currently experiencing greater demand for their services than they have capacity for (i.e., beds available). Policy encourages hospital staff to respond to this issue via efficiency measures rather than expanding capacity. Research shows that displaying art in hospitals reduces pain and decreases recovery time (Lankston et al., 2010; Nielsen et al., 2017; Eminovic et al., 2021). Consequently, by making an upfront investment into artistic displays, hospital commissioners can seek to benefit from long-term reductions in the time that patients spend in their care, thereby increasing their overall capacity.

Medium Impact – With an increased budget, hospital art can be transformed from a still experience to one which encourages physical activity. This is achieved through an arts trail. Here, patients are provided with maps of where core art pieces appear around a hospital, and art is displayed similarly to how it would appear in an art gallery or museum. Jo McAulay, one of the co-designers of Nottingham NHS Trust's art trails comments, 'People have been active whilst exploring the trails, with most walking for between 15 and 30 min whilst exploring the art works. This is hugely important, as physical activity is a factor in both prevention of- and recovery from- illness' (Nottingham Hospitals Charity, 2023). Consequently, from this medium impact provision, hospital patients benefit from reduced pain, decreased recovery time, reduced boredom, and reduced likelihood of future health difficulties.

High Impact – Whilst art and arts trails have the capacity for quality impact on patients, they risk not being interacted with in the absence of a facilitator or guide. Comparatively, participatory arts provisions bring the art to the patients and allow them to be more active participants in the creation of- or enjoyment of- artistic outputs. Participatory arts are able to replicate the type of mental stimulation that a patient would more naturally have access to outside of a clinical environment. They provide a space for joy and reprieve, a method of distraction, and an opportunity to connect with others. Consequently, they not only impact reductions in pain, decreased recovery time, and reduced boredom, but also have significant impacts on mental health, improve relationships between patients and healthcare providers, and improve the likelihood of people accessing care when a problem arises rather than allowing a health issue to develop into an expensive condition to avoid a hospital stay. Adding to this, participatory arts have been shown to impact mutual recovery between patients and healthcare providers

> (Crawford et al., 2013; Hearst, 2024). As workforce wellbeing continues to increase in importance within hospital systems, this can be an effective means of improving mental health and wellbeing without negatively affecting the working capacity of hospital staff. This is particularly helpful in supporting staff who continue to carry the guilt of moral injury, caused throughout the COVID-19 pandemic, instead rebuilding their connection to patients' joy and their sense of self as a helping person.

Here, you can see that scale is clearly demonstratable without the use of a numerical scale. This descriptive language can be used both with or without the supplement of statistics gathered from research outputs, allowing new innovations to be freely promoted and accessed. This clarity of scale provides commissioners with a clear sense of how their investment impacts different areas of health, depending on the budgets they allocate, thereby improving their ability to make an informed decision despite not holding expertise in Creative Health.

The Use of a Descriptive Scale in User-Centred Promotions

To demonstrate how the language of scale might appear within promotional materials, I provide one final illustrative example. This example is based on a hypothetical Creative Health provision, for means of demonstration. Within this example, the problem being addressed is the emotional distress that results from processing trauma. The scale I am indicating is that the service is a supportive mechanism rather than a service which tackles trauma narratives themselves:

> Are you currently on a journey of healing from trauma? Whether you are accessing counselling services or using self-help tools to better understand yourself, we are here to help you manage the distressing emotions that this process can elicit.
>
> Our immersive music display provides a relaxing environment for you to process your feelings and regulate your body's response to distress. Within the room, participants are provided with a space of their own to harness a feeling of safety and solitude. Our live and relaxing music is coupled with soft lighting, slow moving abstract animations, and aromatic smells to create a stimulation-light experience which offers a reprieve from the busy outside world.

As you can see in this example, this promotional communication does not only describe the provision that is available, but it also contextualises it within a particular mental health journey. For members of the public who might feel apprehensive about going to therapy or beginning a trauma-related journey of healing, this communication addresses the whole picture. I believe this style of communication may be particularly of use within public health agendas, to increase mental health literacy in the public and use this as a tool for encouraging more preventative self-care or service interaction.

Final Thoughts...

Throughout this chapter I have described a number of ways that the language of scale can improve communication with service-users, research participants, and commissioners. Through these examples, I have attempted to demonstrate also the importance of creative exploration activities, tiered negotiations, and mental health literacy in the improvement of mental health and wellbeing support. This shows how a single tool of communication can be used in a variety of ways. Accordingly, I invite you to explore the Scale of Impact further, in your own personal or professional contexts, to uncover other outcomes of its use. It is through this ongoing innovation and collaborative thought that we will develop as a Creative Health sector and have our work valued for everything it is worth.

References

Aje (2022) Interview with Jane Hearst.

Crawford, P. et al. (2013) Creative practice as mutual recovery in mental health. *Mental Health Review Journal*, 18(2), pp. 55–64.

Eminovic, S. et al. (2021) Positive effect of colors and art in patient rooms on patient recovery after total hip or knee arthroplasty: A randomized controlled trial. *Wiener klinische Wochenschrift*, [Online] Available at: https://doi.org/10.1007/s00508-021-01936-6 [Accessed 26/01/2022].

Hearst, J. (2024) *Workforce Wellbeing and Cultural Change, via Creative Health.* [Online] National Centre for Creative Health | News and Blogs. Available at: https://ncch.org.uk/blog/workforce-wellbeing-and-cultural-change-via-creative-health [Accessed 04/07/2024].

Lankston, L. et al. (2010) Visual art in hospitals: Case studies and review of the evidence. *Journal of the Royal Society of Medicine*, 103(12), pp. 490–499.

Nielsen, S.L. et al. (2017) How do patients actually experience and use art in hospitals? The significance of interaction: A user-oriented experimental case study. *International Journal of Qualitative Studies on Health and Well-being*, 12(1), p. 1267343.

Nottingham Hospitals Charity (2023) *New Arts Trails Launch at Nottingham Hospitals*. Available at: https://www.nottinghamhospitalscharity.org.uk/news/new-arts-trails-launch-at-nottingham-hospitals [Accessed 03/07/2024].

Samawah (2022) Interview with Jane Hearst.

Chapter 11

Wellbeing Orientations

The question explored in this chapter also draws upon an activity which has been discussed earlier in this book. The Seven Orientations (7O) activity that I used to interact with members of the public, during the co-design on this framework, provided the bedrock of information collected from their stories. The categories demonstrated their usefulness as a data-collection device and were then evaluated as being useful frames of reference within this Creative Health Communication Framework. However, the orientations used within this framework are more advanced than those used within data collection, as they have been developed via participant feedback, to create the Advanced Model of Wellbeing Orientation (Figure 11.1).

Tier One: Ability to Orientate

Functioning in a tiered system, this Advanced Model of Wellbeing Orientation first asks service-providers to discern whether their users have an ability to orientate. **Ability to Orientate** describes barriers to orientation that a person has little control over. Particularly useful considerations within this category are whether a person:

1 has lost retention of some their core or short-term memories
2 cannot distinguish between that which is real and imaginary
3 experiences challenges associated with a neurodivergent mind
4 has an over-active fight-flight-or-freeze response due to trauma
5 is discriminated against in ways that cause barriers to living

These barriers can have an isolating affect between the individual and the external world. For this reason, services that support a user's ability to orientate may focus on reducing the impact of this barrier.

There may be other obstacles that individuals identify within this category in addition to the five listed above, which are more unique to them. These five describe specialist forms of care, which are built upon barriers shared across

DOI: 10.4324/9781003423317-16

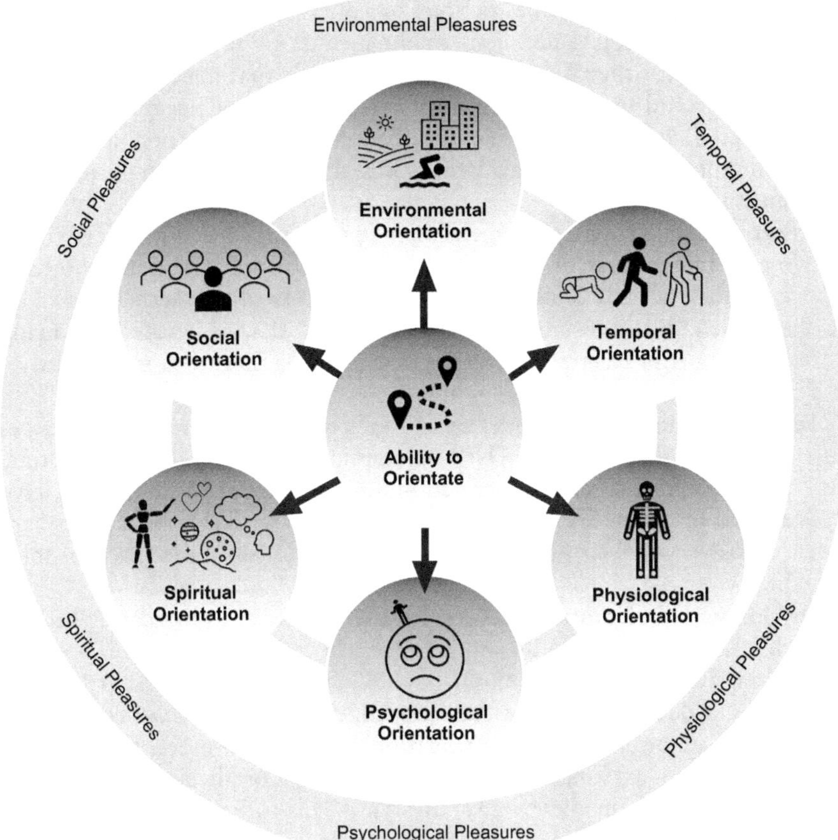

Figure 11.1 The Advanced Model of Wellbeing Orientation.

a demographic. Consequently, services may feature demographics within their promotional communication as they are central to the design of the service. The specificity of these needs may lead to Creative Health support services being described as interventions, as there is often a clear and measurable outcome that the service intends to support.

Tier Two: Wellbeing Orientations

If a service-user is not struggling with a disabling barrier to wellbeing, but instead experiencing an absence of well-aligned resources, then the other six orientations provide a context through which service-providers can bring clarity into their promotional language.

Social Orientation describes actions or values which take place within a service-user's social life. This might include things like their sense of belonging, or their access to a tribe of people that make them feel special. It could include loneliness, having a voice, being understood, or accepted. It might even include their ability to interpret non-verbal communication, or societal pressures that shape who they feel they must be.

Environmental Orientation might include physical aspects of the environment, like a service-user's access to sunlight and whether they have enough space to conduct activities in. Or it might be something more complex, like the emotional environment that is created by being around people who are ill, depressed, grieving, negative, manipulative, abusive, or simply lacking in hope.

Temporal Orientation includes disruptions to plans, like many of us experienced during the COVID-19 pandemic. These factors might be time pressures from a service-user's community, such as expectations to have a child or get married soon. It could involve work-life balance, where one aspect of their life begins to dominate. Or even the speed of their lifestyle.

Physiological Orientation asks service-users about the physical sensations that impact their wellbeing. It might be symptoms they experience when they are stressed, anxious, or having a panic attack. Alternatively, it could describe the pain they hold in their chest when they are processing emotional distress or heartache. For some users, they may be living through a long-standing illnesses, aches, or physical impairments that affect their day-to-day lifestyle. This orientation could even describe sadness related to the appearance of the physical body, as experienced by people with gender dysphoria or body dysmorphia.

Spiritual Orientation describes aspects of a service-user's life which help them to feel connected to the wider world and offer them a sense of meaning. It can include the values that motivate them and guide their actions or a type of work that they thrive in. These may be religious aspects of their life or things in their imagination that help them to feel connected to the planet. This can include calming or sensory activities that ground them when life gets chaotic.

Psychological Orientation differs from the other orientations as it is more likely to consider wellbeing factors which come from within the service-user, such as an internal dialogue that makes an otherwise harmless interaction feel overwhelming. Factors in this orientation can include traumatic memories that trigger an internal response, or insecurities which ruin a service-user's day. Some may seek support because they have developed a set of damaging emotional patterns that they can't break away from.

Tier Three: Pleasures

For service-users who experience a high baseline of wellbeing, they may not require support with either disabling barriers or areas of disorientation. In this case, the service-provider likely has the purpose of maintaining wellbeing or eliciting joyful emotions. These elements move beyond supporting a person in their ability to survive, towards helping them on their mission to thrive. For participants in my research, this aspect of wellbeing was best described as 'pleasure.' Like the orientations, pleasures can be distinguished across six categories: Social Pleasures, Environmental Pleasures, Temporal Pleasures, Physiological Pleasures, Spiritual Pleasures, and Physiological Pleasures. This distinction between wellbeing orientation and pleasures was one that was created by the members of the public that co-designed the Creative Health Communication Framework. They thought that it was important to distinguish fun-focused activity from that which has a more formal or serious wellbeing focus.

Why Speak in Terms of Orientation?

The orientations are particularly useful in assisting a user-provider team to compartmentalise different aspects of a user's wellbeing and identify what types of disorientation they are experiencing. By utilising this tool within communications with service-users, service-providers can be clear about which aspect of a user's experience they are able to contribute to and which aspects are best assisted by collaborating support services. The act of breaking wellbeing down into clearer categories can offer service-users clarity, which, in turn, reduces the likelihood that service-users:

1 misunderstand what aspect of their wellbeing providers can support
2 wrongfully assume that a service can help their entire wellbeing
3 feel too unclear about how a service will achieve success to bother taking part

By utilising the orientations as reference points within discussions, even deviations away from these labels become useful for service-providers to better understand the way that service-users perceive their wellbeing.

Inherent within these orientation descriptors is the understanding that multiple forms of disorientation can occur at the same time within different categories. During moments of combined distress, service-users are likely to feel overwhelmed. For some, they may be very aware of their poor wellbeing but are either too exhausted to think about the co-existing stressors or have too many things to think about at once to be able to target one at a time. This is where a service-provider proves particularly useful in supporting their journey, removing the cognitive burden of service-users to filter or unveil the complexities of their experience. Alternatively, for service-users who have a clear concept of what they hope to change, it can be comforting to access service-providers who are equally clear about the intentions of their service and it reduces the energy required of them to identify a suitable support service.

Another reason why the orientations prove important is to reduce selection bias. Selection bias is where a person's pre-conceived notions (in this case, of wellbeing) distort the way that others' experiences are perceived (in this case, service-users). Based on my observation of current market promotions, service-providers appear to believe that they hold a shared conceptualisation of wellbeing with their service-users. This conceptualisation may be based on their own experience of wellbeing, knowledge learnt through literature or videos, or their perception of normative ways of being. By using the Advanced Model of Wellbeing Orientation as a guide, service-providers are made more aware of the distinctive elements of wellbeing that might be at play, and can, therefore, reduce the risk of selection bias. Bias is reduced because the user can clearly signal where their understandings align or deviate from the orientation labels, rather than using language that has different meanings to different people. Moreover, by segmenting a wellbeing experience into co-existing challenges and emotional states, a service-provider and their users are better able to replicate the complexity of real-life, rather than treat wellbeing like a single unified experience.

Examples from Participants' Stories

To demonstrate the distinction between wellbeing orientations and pleasures more clearly, and to demonstrate the usefulness of the Advanced Model of Wellbeing Orientation, I will provide an overview of two key examples from my interviews with members of the public.

The first example comes from Ekundayo (2021) who used the orientations to discuss their complex experience of 'family.' In their emotional environment, Ekundayo described how the abuse from one of their parents overwhelmed the feelings they associated with home and their life at the time. This deteriorated their psychological wellbeing, as it made them feel suicidal.

Their siblings, on the other hand, provided Ekundayo with a sense of togetherness; a form of spiritual meaning that gave them the strength to survive through the abuse. Once Ekundayo left their parents' house and had their first child, they recognised a power shift, whereby they were now the parent who got to choose values to instil. This provided them with another type of spiritual wellbeing; a protective factor that has considerably changed their life thereafter (Ekundayo, 2021). By presenting the story in this way, Ekundayo was able to conclude that the presence of strong spiritual orientation, via positive family associations, acted as a necessary protective mechanism against their more toxic experiences of family. A service-provider, in this type of scenario, may wish to support changes in Ekundayo's environment and psychology over the long-term, whilst appreciating the importance of prioritising the maintenance of their spiritual orientation along the way.

The second example comes from Devan (2021) who was one of the participants who promoted the distinction between wellbeing orientations and pleasures. They said:

> I've got osteoarthritis in my left knee now. But I can dance for a bit and sit down and then chair dance for a bit and then dance a bit more. And it's about pacing and finding that balance and still enjoying music.

Here, Deven used 'wellbeing' to refer to their management of osteoarthritis on a day-to-day basis – how frequently or to what extent it affects their ability to feel well. Whereas music and dance represented Devan's hobbies and passions. Devan built upon the lessons of managing their condition day-to-day, in the search for specific moments of creative bliss (Devan, 2021). This distinction between wellbeing and joy can be an important feature in engaging specific audiences towards Creative Health provisions. By allowing elements of creativity to remain in the domain of pleasure and self-led activity, rather than speak of them in terms of health-promoting activity and services, individuals are provided greater autonomy to engage with Creative Health on their own terms. The role of service-providers is to recognise where they are situated in these distinctions and how that affects the relational dynamics they will experience with those who engage in their services.

In addition to these specific examples, I have chosen to provide a short list of bullet points demonstrating the type of elements that featured in participants' stories when discussing positive orientation factors. These factors have been selected based on what participants labelled as highly influential parts of their story during the Scale of Influence activity. They are not intended to be an exhaustive list of factors which fall under each category, rather a springboard for ideas and an indicator of where protective factors may be placed.

Social:

- Good upbringing and access to quality education
- Compatible chosen family
- Friends/tribes that encourage good decisions
- Friends/tribes that foster uplifting values
- Freedom from judgement and harmful competitiveness

- A sense of belonging at the societal level
- The people that are seen regularly foster a positive environment
- Freedom from unfit systemised pressures (e.g., misaligned cultural practices)
- A unit from which one can derive a sense of purpose (e.g., a family)
- Places that facilitate group learning, experimentation, and socialising
- Acceptance of the self in all its forms (e.g., through various styles of socialising)

Psychological:

- Moments that put life into perspective and the ability to adapt around them
- The ability to maintain internal strength through moments of change and vulnerability
- A space to release emotions and the bravery to do so
- Prioritisation of self-care above damaging social pressures
- Making the choice to practise healthy habits
- Freedom from depression and its debilitating effects
- An awareness of what 'my best' means in the present day, and a freedom from outdated versions of the self
- Ability to withstand the internalisation of toxicity from negative people and practices around us
- Relationships that support our sense of self rather than erode it
- Inspiration to achieve and live out one's passions and purpose despite strain
- Cultivate a positive sense of self and ritualistically communicate to- and reflect on- this self

Physiological:

- Manageable responsibility in terms of energy and activity offered to others
- Manageable levels of stress
- Absence of chronic pain
- Absence from anxiety or panic and their distressing physiological symptoms
- A healthy emotional relationship with the physical self

Environmental:

- Work that is enjoyed
- A country that is a pleasure to be in
- Strong and healthy relationships
- Activities that engage with meaning and promote personal skill or worth

- Freedom from emotional and physical abuse
- A comfortable, safe, and social home
- Access to play
- Control and choice over the people one comes in contact with
- Happy and healthy loved ones
- Clean and green spaces

Spiritual:

- A reason to be alive which outweighs the pressures that put this in doubt
- A sense of purpose, or responsibilities, that are within our reach
- Ability to practise mindfulness on one's own
- Access to role models or counterparts that provide a sense of meaning
- Ability to explore, witness, and learn from different communities and places
- Be able to give, receive, and develop love – for self and for others

Temporal:

- Work which does not overtake life
- Financial security and the temporal freedom it provides

Applying the Learning to Creative Health

Different Creative Health services are naturally well aligned to different types of orientation. By making references to these orientations, Creative Health practitioners can demonstrate the strengths that differentiate them from traditional medical services. Moreover, where multiple Creative Health provisions are able to contribute to the same orientation-limiting health concern, this frame invites stakeholders to identify their unique selling point in what they can support. To demonstrate, I will provide some key examples.

In the category of Ability to Orientate, a fantastic example coming from the research literature is the place of Creative Health in supporting those with dementia and other neurological conditions. The role that Creative Health can play in the support of dementia patients is rich and can derive from a range of creative methods. These include having a positive effect on attention and stimulation of memories (Young, Camic and Tischler, 2016), improving verbal fluency, and reducing anxiety, depression, and apathy (Lam et al., 2020), as well as supporting better working memory and improved executive function/language (Bone et al., 2022). The arts also play a role in better researching and understanding experiences of dementia (Camic et al., 2021; Harding et al., 2021), so that more proficient care systems can be designed. Moreover, they can play a preventative role. For example, 'social networks and social participation have [...] been shown to act as protective factors against dementia or cognitive decline over the age of 65' (Allen and Allen, 2016), and participatory arts are often inherently social. The financial value of dementia-focused Creative Health provisions is also demonstrable. For example, investors can expect up to £6.62 Social Return on Investment for every £1 invested in visual arts interventions for dementia (Jones, Windle and Edwards, 2018) and £149 million is saved annually, thanks to how movement and dance reduce the risk of developing dementia (Boardman et al., 2023). These services each support or prevent people who are living with a potentially isolating and confusing condition, maintaining as much independence as possible and ensuring that those without that independence can still experience a life which is rich and joyful.

Elsewhere, Creative Health services can support a wide range of wellbeing orientations. One great example of this, coming from the sector, is Queer Black Christmas. Queer Black Christmas is a 'celebration for Black LGBTQ+ young people from London, who are experiencing homelessness, living in temporary accommodation or in hostile home environments' (Compas, 2023). This is one of many events hosted by Existing Loudly, a grassroots organisation 'committed to creating spaces of joy, community and care for Black LGBTQ+ youth from London through creative intervention' (Compas, 2020). Their aim 'is to recreate a Christmas where Black LGBTQ+ youth can bring their full selves to the dinner table, a Christmas where they can feel like kids again, a Christmas where they are allowed to just exist.' Inherent in this service is a focus on social orientation – supporting Black LGBTQIA+ young people going through hardship to find others who experience their own intersections, so that their sense of self can be affirmed and their community expanded. In addition to this, a key focus of Queer Black Christmas is temporal orientation – both because this is a space created at Christmas time, when many LGBTQIA+ youth experience an increase in hostility or discrimination from the family unit or feel more isolated due to the focus on familial celebration, and because one of the target audiences for the service are those experiencing the precariousness of temporary accommodation. Implicit in the support being offered here is an acknowledgement that, without a safe space like this to celebrate, Black LGBTQIA+ young people are at risk of serious decline in their mental health. Research has shown that acute distress relating to discrimination, concealment, and/or rejection sensitivity causes LGBTQIA+ individuals to be at higher risk of 'internalising' mental health disorders (Eaton, 2020; Eaton, Rodriguez-Seijas and Pachankis, 2021). This act of internalising leaves LGBTQIA+ individuals at increased risk of depression, suicide, and substance use, compared to their cis-gender, heterosexual counterparts (Mongelli et al., 2019). Consequently, the social and temporal benefits of Queer Black Christmas are significant and worthy of more attention from health commissioners.

As a final example, I can compare Queer Black Christmas to another socially motivated community provision – a samba drumming band. This example comes from my own experience of taking part in a group called

Sambando in Leicester. Here, the social connection derived from the activity is more often considered one of pleasure. This is not because there is an absence of links between group music playing and mental health, in fact, playing in a samba band is a fantastic way of boosting the chemicals in our brains which are associated with group bonding (Tarr, Launay and Dunbar, 2014). It also develops communal language systems, such as the call and response feature of group music playing (Wöllner, 2020). However, despite the potential benefits this group has on mental health and wellbeing, it is not promoted as a wellbeing service, nor do the leaders of the group intend to take any responsibility for the mental health of its participants. The attendees go to this group to supplement their wellbeing with social pleasure, helping them to remain well rather than become well.

Final Thoughts...

The exact wording that service-providers use in their promotional communication is unlikely to refer to orientation directly, as this language is very formal and describes a particular theory which the user may not be aware of. But by using these orientations as a probing mechanism, service-providers can gain a clearer idea of the orientation they predominantly seek to impact and where, within it, their service lies. From this guidance grows opportunity for creative expression and innovation.

References

Allen, J. and Allen, M. (2016) The social determinants of health, empowerment, and participation. In: Clift, S. and Camic, P.M. (eds.) *Oxford Textbook of Creative Arts, Health, and Wellbeing: International Perspectives on Practice, Policy, and Research*. Oxford Textbooks in Public Health. Oxford, United Kingdom: Oxford University Press, pp. 27–34.

Boardman, R. et al. (2023) *Social Value of Movement and Dance*. London: Sport + Recreation Alliance.

Bone, J.K. et al. (2022) Participatory and receptive arts engagement in older adults: Associations with cognition over a seven-year period. PsyArXiv. https://doi.org/10.1080/10400419.2023.2217211

Camic, P.M. et al. (2021) Developing poetry as a research methodology to further understand rarer forms of dementia. In: *Culture, Health and Wellbeing International Conference (CHW21) Research Proceedings. Culture, Health and Wellbeing International Conference (CHW21)*. UK: Arts and Health South West.

Compas, T. (2020) *Homepage – Existing Loudly*. [Online] Instagram. Available at: https://www.instagram.com/existloudly/?hl=en [Accessed 12/08/2023].

Compas, T. (2023) *What is Queer Black Christmas*. [Online] Existing Loudly. Available at: https://ww2.emma-live.com/existloudly/?pageview&page=about+-queer+black+christmas [Accessed 12/08/2023].

Devan (2021) Interview with Jane Hearst.

Eaton, N.R. (2020) Measurement and mental health disparities: Psychopathology classification and identity assessment. *Personality and Mental Health*, 14(1), pp. 76–87.

Eaton, N.R., Rodriguez-Seijas, C. and Pachankis, J.E. (2021) Transdiagnostic approaches to sexual- and gender-minority mental health. *Current Directions in Psychological Science*, 30(6), pp. 510–518.

Ekundayo (2021) Interview with Jane Hearst.

Harding, E. et al. (2021) Developing a drawing-based method to capture and communicate experiences of rare dementias. In: *Culture, Health and Wellbeing International Conference (CHW21) Research Proceedings. Culture, Health and Wellbeing International Conference (CHW21)*. UK: Arts and Health South West.

Jones, C., Windle, G. and Edwards, R.T. (2018) Dementia and imagination: A social return on investment analysis framework for art activities for people living with dementia. *The Gerontologist*, [Online] Available at: https://doi.org/10.1093/geront/gny147 [Accessed 13/12/2023].

Lam, H.L. et al. (2020) Effects of music therapy on patients with dementia—A systematic review. *Geriatrics*, 5(4), p. 62.

Mongelli, F. et al. (2019) Minority stress and mental health among LGBT populations: an update on the evidence. *Minerva Psichiatrica*, 60(1), [Online] Available at: https://doi.org/10.23736/S0391-1772.18.01995-7 [Accessed 22/11/2022].

Tarr, B., Launay, J. and Dunbar, R.I.M. (2014) Music and social bonding: 'Self-other' merging and neurohormonal mechanisms. *Frontiers in Psychology*, 5, [Online] Available at: https://doi.org/10.3389/fpsyg.2014.01096 [Accessed 28/10/2024].

Wöllner, C. (2020) Call and response: Musical and bodily interactions in jazz improvisation duos. *Musicae Scientiae*, 24(1), pp. 44–59.

Young, R., Camic, P.M. and Tischler, V. (2016) The impact of community-based arts and health interventions on cognition in people with dementia: A systematic literature review. *Aging & Mental Health*, 20(4), pp. 337–351.

Chapter 12

Absent or Misaligned Resources

In Chapters 6 and 8, I commented on MacKinnon & Derickson's (2013) critique of resilience, which suggests that poorly designed systems of power can have an erosive effect on wellbeing. Within this theme, I describe how systematic voices can conflict with a service-user's voice and can, therefore, be considered an unfit resource. This, coupled with stories from participant interviews, led to the development of the theme that is central to this chapter – the absence/loss of resources versus misaligned resources. This theme challenges normative conceptions about mental health services, as it does not assume that those requiring help are people who lack. Rather it demonstrates that, at times, individuals can have access to resources and societal guidance, yet feel held back by the incompatibility of these resources. Moreover, in instances where individuals do lack resources, this can be due to systematic discrimination and structures rather than a character flaw. By allowing for all these nuances and possibilities, we reduce the stigma associated with accessing support and guidance, hence why it is important to consider in our communication about mental health and wellbeing.

Distinguishing Absent and Misaligned Resources

Absent or lost resources describe a scenario when an individual lacks the physical or mental assets that help them to manage their emotions or reach their goals. A good example of this came from within Samawah's interview where they said 'I know what can be done to help me in the situation that I am [in] and become a better version of me. It's just that I don't have the resources' (Samawah, 2022).

Misaligned resources, on the other hand, describe something which is considered an asset by others, even though it conflicts with the values or goals of the individual who possesses this asset. For this reason, these 'assets' might feel like a burden; they create a barrier to accessing support, as the individual is not without resources, yet the misalignment of these resources

DOI: 10.4324/9781003423317-17

can prove very isolating and dissatisfying. A good example of a participant who undertook a journey of abandoning misaligned resources in search of better-fitting resources is Kris. Kris made the decision to move from a prestigious profession towards a more meaningful passion, despite the cultural pressures to be in a 'respectable' job (Kris, 2021). They said, 'I'd gone from a two-bedroom, semi-detached house with a double driveway with my ex, in [a big UK city], to sleeping in a box room at my grand[parent]'s with all my stuff in a loft' (Kris, 2021). Making this change towards better aligned resources took great strength, as Kris had to endure the discomfort of disassembling misaligned resources whilst cultivating appropriate resources in their replacement. The type of support they required was not in accessing resources but in helping them to maintain strength during this difficult transition.

The distinction between these two types of wellbeing struggles is particularly important in addressing some of the inherent presumptions of the market. Namely, many service-users hold the presumption that they should only access mental health services, such as counselling, when they are experiencing an absence of resources or when trauma has caused internal deterioration (see Chapter 9 for details). An issue that arises when wellbeing is treated this way is that for people who have not experienced major/self-evident traumas or those who have access to many resources but not the ones they need, there is a stigma associated with accessing care. Through this stigma, individuals are more likely to perceive their problem as not being big enough to be worthy of care. For example, within Aje's interview, they shared that they struggled with feelings of guilt and uncertainty when they chose to continue counselling, as it was difficult to put some of the responsibility on somebody else, especially when Aje felt that they didn't need it enough to warrant that allocation of responsibility (Aje, 2022). Similarly, some individuals in this situation fear that by engaging with a service, they could be taking resources from someone with more clear traumas, or that their involvement in this service might signal to others that they are victims rather than people in pursuit of self-actualisation.

As I explored in Chapter 9, complex wrongdoing – the type associated with self-actualisation – can be equally or more damaging than clear wrongdoings, such as abuse-related traumas. Consequently, to have a mental wellbeing market that prioritises the care of clear wrongdoings over complex wrongdoings can be considered unjust. Only by expanding our knowledge of misaligned resources and the way they affect the individual can this deficit of the market be adequately responded to. Once this knowledge is acquired, service-providers are better positioned to communicate their ability to support service-users who are struggling with misaligned resources and reduce the stigmas that exist in the market at present.

Personal versus Systematic Misalignment

Within participant stories there were two distinct types of resource misalignment. The first is personal and unique to the individual, a great example being the dominant environment that individuals find themselves in. The second is systematic misalignments. These describe dominant social frameworks in which large groups of people are asked to abide by, despite whether they work in their favour or not. To demonstrate, I will refer a selection of participant examples. The first comes from Jiva, who discussed the benefits of changing their dominant environment.

Following Jiva's involvement in a competitive sport, they craved the adrenaline rush that they used to experience. The social circle that they were drawn to was made up of people who had lots of money – much of which was spent on drugs and alcohol. The highs of this lifestyle filled a void for Jiva, but it led to addictive behaviours and an involvement in crime. Then, one day, Jiva was placed in jail (Jiva, 2022). In our interview, Jiva said, 'At that time, I was heavily into the drugs [...] so it just cleared my head completely [...] [it was] probably the best holiday I ever had' (Jiva, 2022). Jiva explained that going to jail helped them to escape from some of their addictive behaviours and completely remove themselves from criminal social circles. Motivating this change was Jiva's guiding thought: 'jail's for jokers, not for me' (Jiva, 2022).

In Jiva's story, they described their old social circle as a misaligned resource, as even though they could offer Jiva the adrenalin rushes they craved, they also encouraged Jiva to partake in crime, excessive alcohol intake, and the illegal consumption of drugs (Jiva, 2022). This is an example of personal misalignment. Here, the communities that Jiva accessed can be considered 'resources' as they affect Jiva's wellbeing. Once this resource was identified as being misaligned, Jiva was more able to seek out communities that were representative of how Jiva wanted to live their life and improve their wellbeing in the process.

Elsewhere in participant interviews, people identified aspects of national cultures that either aligned or misaligned. Ngoen (2022), for example, spoke to me about improvements they experienced after moving to the UK. They had a long list of positive qualities they could attribute to the UK, including forgiving work environments, clean and green streets, respect for authority, convenient transportation, animal welfare, ability to have savings, and lack of hazards in their physical space. Ngoen contrasted these positives to the lasting impression they took from Thailand, whereby toxicity was at the core of their narrative. Ngoen defined toxicity as 'the willingness to eat each other up, but not going anywhere' (Ngoen, 2022), saying that, in Thailand, they were surrounded by people who just lived to judge. Moreover, they explained that the amount of energy that they put in was not equal to what they gained, highlighting the importance of having minimum standards of living, as afforded in the UK.

But whilst Ngoen described an improvement in wellbeing thanks to moving to the UK, the country is not without its own problems. In Devan's interview, they compared the UK now to how it was in the past, and identified a reduction in living standards:

> My hope for the future is that we can dramatically swing back – somewhere like Britain 30–40 years [ago] – to have a different political thing [...] I'd like to see a more equitable, more tolerant, more just society in Britain [...] I'm very cynical about that. So, my plan B is that, if that's not going to happen in the next five years or so, I'll probably move.
>
> (Devan, 2021)

Two of Devan's main reasons for upholding this position were related to the working culture of the UK and an increased lack of community (Devan, 2021).

Misaligned resources can have a tremendously negative affect on an individual when they are experienced at the level of society as these environments are inescapable. Ngoen and Devan both referenced moving to a different country to escape from misaligned values, but this is not always possible for different individuals. This demonstrates just how important it is to recognise misalign resources and address them, particularly when they belong to large systems that are largely out of the control of an individual.

Systematic Voices versus the Abstraction of the Arts

Through participant interviews, we identified numerous distinct systems which have attempted to influence the life choices of different participants. These included cultural, spiritual, intellectual, popular, financial, technological, moral, political, and community voices. As you can see in Figure 12.1, these voices were drawn from systems in the external world and were then personalised by the individual who negotiated the purpose and priority of different systems within their lives.

Based on participant data, I conceive that what individuals deliver back into the world is a more creative voice; one which reconceptualises rigid values and innovates around the unique needs that they have experienced. The state of these pathways between internal and external worlds – that is, the degree of equity – has been shown throughout participants interviews to determine a great deal regarding their wellbeing. Where there is synchronicity, affirmation is achieved. Where there is conflict, there is potential for the individual to feel powerless and othered. In the first scenario, the individual is able to attain internal abundance (see Chapter 9 for more details), whereas the latter scenario inevitably leads toward internal deterioration.

The importance of this concept of voices, for Creative Health researchers and service-providers, is the state of the *individual's* voice. Since this is the

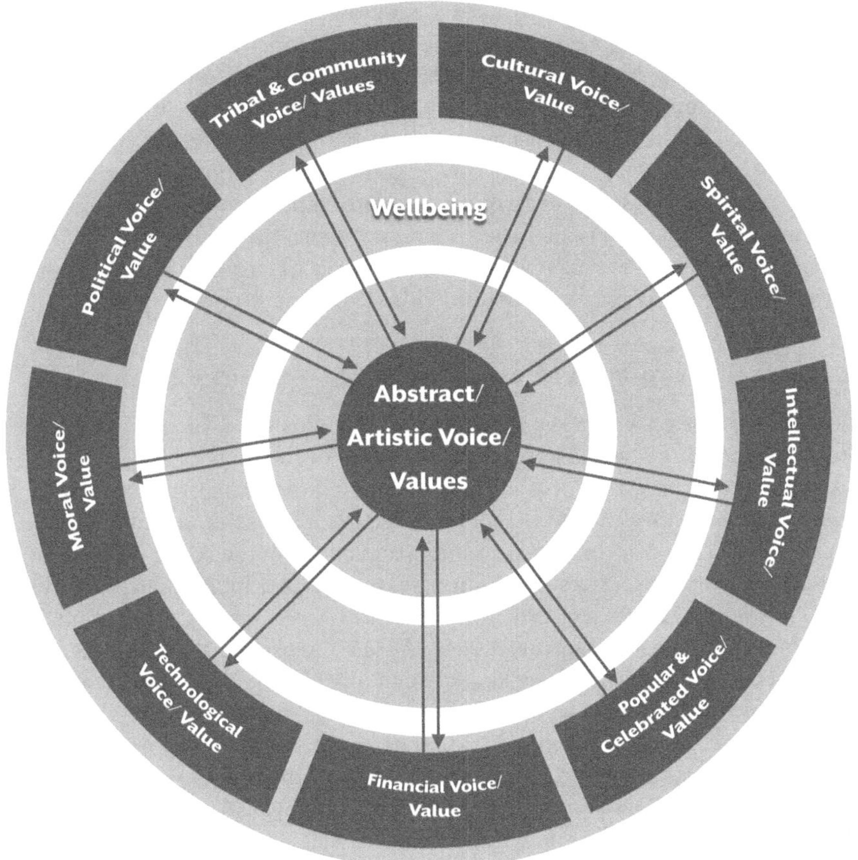

Figure 12.1 The interrelation of systematic and individual 'voices' within value negotiation.

voice that negotiates the demands of different systems, via a personal perception of value, it can be seen to be far more creative than the rigid structures of systematised voices. The flexibility of this creative voice is, therefore, compatible with the abstract nature of artistic philosophies. By engaging with artistic practices, the abstract voice can be nurtured and given more power – at least at the level of the individual – and this abstract voice can offer service-users an opportunity for reprieve.

Within its abstraction, artistic practice grants space for service-users to celebrate a range of different ways of knowing, celebrating voices of intricacy, fallibility, rebellious innovation, and playful simplicity. These expressions may form movements of institutional protest, facilitate tribe-based connection, or act simply as a means of catharsis, embracing the chaos that is value negotiation. This acknowledgement of the self, as a reflection of imperfectly negotiated values, allows individuals to strip away their outer social shells and imagine a world in which their inner self exists separate to these external forces. Once an internal world has been cultivated to inhabit authentic values and their associated joy, service-providers can then refocus their efforts back on the absence of resource in the external world. This return to the external might involve the individual repositioning their life within new systems or environments that support their sense of self. Alternatively, it may involve the individual using the arts to communicate difficult or non-verbal concepts to people in their external world, in the hope of connecting these people to the individual's internal world.

Considering the Market as a Misaligned Resource

A systematic voice which is particularly vital to this book's investigation into 'market wellbeing' (see Chapter 6), is the voice of the marketplace and all the social/financial pressures this entails. These pressures distort the balance of daily experience and can *cause* mental ill-health. This is important as Creative Health services may experience limitations if they seek market funding towards wellbeing services that support issues *caused* by market pressures.

In participant interviews, the topic of the capitalist market was implicit in a number of stories. During Lou's (2021) interview, for example, they expressed relief that they worked in their profession during an era where human connection was able to flourish. They explained that things are becoming increasingly automated and that, in the parts of the job that do still involve humans, there are separated workstations, so current employees don't have the camaraderie that they used to. Lou believes these automations were money-motivated. Likewise, in Gayle's (2021) interview, they echoed these concerns. Gayle explained that they experienced moments in their live where they survived off very little money, such as during the Second World War, but were able to thrive regardless. They reflected on the values of the present generation and noted that they have many more commercial resources but carry no values of sharing love: 'The values are completely different [...] We don't love one another today, I don't think. [...] It saddens me because although we didn't have as much money as we've got today, we had a better life' (Gayle, 2021).

Within these stories, both Lou and Gayle expressed concern for the deterioration of protective values and their replacement by commercialised gratifications. They reflected over long periods of time and were able to deliver a wide range of stories which illustrated how this deterioration was shaping society and an individual's ability to feel well.

One of the challenges of aligning Creative Health practices to our current marketplace is that many causes of ill wellbeing can be linked to negative consumeristic behaviours and increasingly distorted views that objects and money can solve issues of the heart. This conflict exists between the voice of the market (which is concerned with economic prosperity) and the voice of the service-user (which is concerned with human prosperity). Addressing the problems that arise from these views and behaviours involves the challenging of consumeristic philosophies; something that is in direct opposition to the values of the market. It is for this reason, that Creative Health services that challenge capitalist market ideals tend to struggle with accessing financial support.

My ability to develop a Creative Health Communication is also affected by this conflict of interest and it is through my identification of misaligned resources that I attempt to make this conflict transparent. By providing service-providers with the language of misaligned resources, they are better able to debate the terms of a capitalist market and describe its erosive effects on mental health and wellbeing.

Applying the Learning to Creative Health

Creative Health is able to support individuals with both absent and misaligned resources, it is able to work at both a personal and systematic level, and change can be achieved both via Creative Health activities and Creative Health approaches. Here, I detail two examples to demonstrate.

In my first example I invite you to consider the shortcomings of traditional therapy services in regard to people who are minoritised. LGBTQIA+ people, for example, often feel misunderstood by their counsellors, as their conceptualisation of gender, expressions of identity, community norms, use of language, and experience of minority stress hold distance from normative ways of being and knowing. This can be an isolating experience for those who access a misaligned service, yet it does not mean that talking therapies do not have a place to play in their lives. Julie Tilsen (2021) teaches us how to better align therapy services to the needs of LGBTQIA+ individuals in her book *Queering Your Therapy Practice: Queer Theory, Narrative Therapy, and Imagining New Identities*. In this, Tilsen uses creativity and play techniques to revitalise talking therapies and make them more pertinent to the needs of her clients. An example that she presents in the introductory chapter is the gender unicorn. Here she asks a young non-binary client:

> If the gender Unicorn were to trot in here, burping rainbows and throwing glitter everywhere, and it made the idea of male and female, gay and straight, and all the rules and assumptions that go with these things disappear, what would happen? What would that make possible?

This new questioning technique quickly demonstrated differences in the body language of the client, as well as their creative engagement with thoughts. The example shows how Creative Health activity can positively influence the experience of personal misalignment for LGBTQIA+ individuals.

Minoritised groups can also be subjected to an absence of resources. Take People of Colour (POC) or women, for example. Both of these groups are negatively impacted by a lack of research into how health conditions affect their demographic. In the absence of this information there is an absence of safety, a lack of space for these voices, and inaccurate health guidance. One way of responding to this issue is via Creative Health approaches. This includes values such as co-design, Patient and Public Involvement (PPI), and the re-centring of Lived Experience Experts. A great example of how this type of work might be facilitated involves the use of anti-racism frameworks (Oparah et al., 2021; National Institute for Health and Care Excellence, 2022; Health Innovation Network, 2022; Goings et al., 2023). Creative Health providers have also been shown to be great partners within collaborations, as they can often access communities and individuals who are otherwise deemed 'hard to reach.' Balanced with the support of traditional healthcare professionals who offer different strengths, as per the Creative Health Quality Framework (Willis and Hume, 2023), these more dynamic teams are able to support disenfranchised groups more effectively. Moreover, creative research methods, such as the embroidered sister map technique used by Improving Me and University of Liverpool's Mental Health Research Innovation Centre to explore women's mental health journeys (NCCH, 2024), have proved successful in engaging groups who otherwise might not partake in health research. This shows that both Creative Health approaches and activities have a part to play in reducing systematic issues with resource availability, for things such as quality health research.

Final Thoughts...

In this chapter, I explored the final frame from Stage One of the Creative Health Communication Framework. Stage One demonstrates a wide range of opportunities for researchers and service-providers to develop the clarity of their promotional communication, regarding the 'threats to wellbeing' that they seek to support. Through these demonstrations, I have shown that clarity of promotion is not dependent on the measurements and priorities of the sciences. Instead, Creative Health providers can draw upon their specialist knowledge of their craft and celebrate its unique features. By indicating their perceived purpose within a service-users' journey of wellbeing, researchers and service-providers hold themselves accountable and heighten the rigor associated with their provision. Researchers and service-providers can use this clarity to make the identification of support services easier for their users, which embeds their wellbeing function throughout the customer experience.

In the next four chapters, I detail Stage Two of the framework which demonstrates the many ways that researchers and service-providers can approach the act of supporting a user. In clarifying these methods of support, I help researchers and service-providers to improve their communication, not only to their service-users but also to their funders and research collaborators.

References

Aje (2022) Interview with Jane Hearst.

Devan (2021) Interview with Jane Hearst.

Gayle (2021) Interview with Jane Hearst.

Goings, T.C. et al. (2023) An antiracist research framework: Principles, challenges, and recommendations for dismantling racism through research. *Journal of the Society for Social Work and Research*, 14(1), pp. 101–128.

Health Innovation Network (2022) *Anti-racism toolkit*. South London.

Jiva (2022) Interview with Jane Hearst.

Kris (2021) Interview with Jane Hearst.

Lou (2021) Interview with Jane Hearst.

MacKinnon, D. and Derickson, K.D. (2013) From resilience to resourcefulness: A critique of resilience policy and activism. *Progress in Human Geography*, 37(2), pp. 253–270.

National Institute for Health and Care Excellence (2022) The race equality framework: A practitioners guide for public involvement in research. [online] NIHR. Available at: https://www.nihr.ac.uk/nihr-race-equality-framework [Accessed 04/08/2024].

NCCH (2024) *Huddles*. Available at: https://ncch.org.uk/huddles [Accessed 04/08/2024].

Ngoen (2022) Interview with Jane Hearst.

Oparah, J.C. et al. (2021) Creativity, resilience and resistance: Black Birthworkers' responses to the COVID-19 pandemic. *Frontiers in Sociology*, 6, p. 636029.

Samawah (2022) Interview with Jane Hearst.

Tilsen, J.B. (2021) *Queering Your Therapy Practice: Queer Theory, Narrative Therapy, and Imagining New Identities*. New York, NY: Routledge.

Willis, J. and Hume, V. (2023) *The Creative Health Quality Framework*. Barnsley: Culture, Health and Wellbeing Alliance.

Stage 2

The Role of the Service-Provider

Chapter 13

Identifying or Managing Threats

Once a researcher or service-provider has considered the 'threat to wellbeing' they are seeking to support, via the first four frames of the Creative Health Communication Framework, they are then able to consider their role in the journey of support. The second stage in the framework – explored here in Chapters 13–16 – supports researchers and service-providers in identifying, developing, and communicating their role. The first question in this stage of the framework is: *is the service-provider's role to help identify or manage threats to wellbeing?*

Is the Service-Provider's Role to Help Identify or Manage Threats to Wellbeing?

This question was developed in response to participant stories which expressed confusion or conflict relating to the perceived role of a service-provider. To answer this question readers may hold a role in identifying threats, managing threats, or a mixture of the two.

Identifying threats involves an individual engaging with a service or research project to better understand themselves, the burdens they confront, and the value systems that shape their perceptions of these burdens. This type of service involves taking the service-user's complex experience and breaking it down into more manageable and processable concepts or goals. Some service-users come to a service-provider to help them identify threats because they need a bouncing board for their ideas – psychodynamic therapy is a good example of this. Other service-users seek help from a service-provider because they believe the providers' specialist knowledge can identify threats that the user is unaware of – as is the case in neurodivergent diagnostic assessments.

Within the participant interviews, Ngoen exemplified a person who was interested in identifying areas for improvement. They described their use of a habit-tracker, which involved monitoring things they would like to focus on, with dates alongside them. 'If we can't track something, we can't control it' they explained, listing measures such as how they work on their business,

DOI: 10.4324/9781003423317-19

how they support their joints through exercise, or even how often they use the bathroom (Ngoen, 2022). Ngoen also showed a keenness for learning about health behaviours from others around them, demonstrating the place of identifying support in their life.

Managing threats, on the other hand, describes a situation where a service-user is aware of their problems but is struggling to change them. Here, the role of the service-provider is to help the user to minimise the negative effects of this problem on their wellbeing. This might be provided via concrete resources, such as a safe space to visit, or through the application of specialist knowledge, such as activities that reduce bodily responses to trauma. Sometimes, the role of a managing provider may be to assist the service-user in creating a management plan. This is particularly helpful for people with co-occurring threats to wellbeing, neurodevelopmental barriers, or those who have been taught that their voice does not matter.

An example of how a participant has helped their friend to manage their wellbeing came from Gayle. The night before surgery, Gayle's friend called, scared and close to cancelling. Gayle listened to their concerns, reminded them of their motivations, and provided the supportive push that their friend needed. Recalling their own experience, Gayle said, 'You're going to be in pain, it'll hurt, and you will cry. But you want it done' (Gayle, 2021). After a firm talk, Gayle's friend thanked them for helping them to manage their anxieties. Service-users might receive similar support from hospital therapists or third-sector providers.

The Relationship between Identifying and Managing Threats

There is an inherent relationship between these two distinctions: the better a service-user understands their values, burdens, and goals, the more effectively they can pursue change. Participant data highlights the importance of this understanding, as it helps clarify the specific stage in a person's journey where the service-provider assumes responsibility. Here, I briefly explore why this question is important in relation to safeguarding and stigma.

Earlier in this book, I noted that many Creative Health services promote the value of 'giving voice' to their service-users. Whilst this can be very empowering when given the right platform – especially for demographics that society has taught to be quiet or silent – in other scenarios, silence stems from fear. When an individual uses their voice to identify a problem, it can sometimes be one of their only opportunities to gain management support. This was evident in Ekundayo's interview, where they described a moment when their sibling reported the abuse of their parent (Ekundayo, 2021). In Ekundayo's story, social workers visited the parent and spoke with them privately, but following that conversation, the social workers did not speak with the children nor return to offer any support thereafter.

Ekundayo explained that this experience caused significant feelings of hopelessness and despair, facilitating the ongoing abuse that continued thereafter (Ekundayo, 2021). This is one of the reasons service-providers need to be clear on the limits of what they can offer. If they are unable to support or signpost to support for managing any issues identified, the service-user needs to be aware of this prior to disclosure to manage their expectations and maintain trust. Similarly, for some users, they can manage and endure prior to identifying threats, but upon exposing the breadth of wrongdoing or expressing a desire for change, they can be left in a position of vulnerability. Service-providers do not need to stop this from happening, but they do carry a responsibility to either develop an emergency provision procedure, signpost to aftercare, or be clear ahead of time that this is not something they would be able to support themselves.

Another important consideration regarding the service-provider's role is related to stigma. For some service-users, a barrier to receiving care is the perception that service-providers will assume they know best. For those keen to retain control over their decision-making, this assumption can be highly distressing and prevent them from accessing services with more equal power dynamics. In these scenarios, demonstrating that the service-provider's role is to help users identify their own values, threats, and goals can relieve this pressure.

Another stigma that some individuals carry is the understanding that wellbeing services only exist to identify problems. For individuals who feel they carry a strong awareness of their problems it can be frustrating to engage with a service that holds this purpose. By being clear in their purpose, service-providers who hold a function of assisting with the management of wellbeing threats can demonstrate to these individuals that they differ from identifying services.

Collaborations between Identifying and Managing Partners

To explore the link between identifying and managing threats to wellbeing further, I turn to a prominent example from the participant interviews:

During Aje's early adulthood, their disability progressed, and they lost the ability to walk. Aje was taken to hospital and their lifestyle changed significantly. From losing their friendship group, job, car, and independence, to challenging their sense of worth, purpose, and direction, the disability left a big mark on their life. 'I couldn't control my body so how can I control being understood or accepted,' they thought (Aje, 2022).

Whilst Aje went through a period of great transition, they needed the support of both identifying *and* managing services. The aspects of their experience that Aje needed help identifying were new value systems, a sense of purpose, and friendships which aligned to their new sense of self. Whereas the type of management support they required was linked to their ability to have a fulfilling life despite the barriers of their disability (Aje, 2022).

When talking about the difficulties they were having with their friends, Aje explained 'I thought I was part of a tribe when I wasn't' (Aje, 2022). Accepting that these friendships had been conditional and that these conditions were strongly tied to physical abilities was very disheartening for Aje and they obsessed over proving that they were still worthy (Aje, 2022). Thankfully, Aje gained access to support which identified people in similar circumstances to their own. This led Aje to reflect on their combined sense of worth and make a new, more compatible group of friends (Aje, 2022).

Within Aje's storytelling, they then explained the ways that they managed the barriers caused by their disability. From getting a support worker to assist them in getting around, to having a house and workplace that are accessible and which can facilitate the needs of their friends. Being able to manage the barriers of their condition in this way has impacted their quality of life and wellbeing:

> Quality of life is a big thing to me because I've had to fight for it [...] that could be economically, that could be family-wise, could be work-wise [...] and being independent as much as possible. Like I'm part of... I'm doing something meaningful.
>
> (Aje, 2022)

Through this experience, Aje demonstrated that there is a complex relationship between identifying threats to wellbeing and managing them. Only by readdressing their relationship with their disability, accepting it, and readjusting their expectations of others, could they begin to consider the possibilities of a life in which they thrived despite the barriers of a disability. Recognising these new values was only facilitative of wellbeing when it could be coupled with practical resources and management techniques.

Promoting Identification and Management in Traditional Therapies

For researchers or service-providers who apply this framing to their work, it can be a method for unveiling the philosophy that underpins their approach. To demonstrate this, I refer to two traditional therapies.

Narrative Therapy – The philosophy that informs Narrative Therapy believes that service-users are the experts of their values and desires for their life (Hayward, 2022). The therapy is not goal-orientated, as goals can be an expression of what other people expect from the individual. To safeguard them against harmful social discourse, Narrative Therapy focuses on <u>identifying</u> the individual's values and their legacies within the individual's life (Redstone, 2022). Where a person's narrative is self-depreciating, Narrative Therapists guide their clients to <u>identify</u> an alternative story (Denborough, 2014). Through the <u>identification</u> of the alternative story, users can appreciate the multiplicity of their values and how they are negotiated in daily experiences. Returning to their original narratives, the users are then able to identify whether the motivation for their actions is as negative as they reported or whether they had neglected to consider the importance of a different value. This therapy, therefore, helps the individual to appreciate where negative emotions and behaviours come from. This provides them with the information needed to 1) become prouder of their actions, 2) be more accepting of their fallibility, or 3) reprioritise their values.

CBT Informed Anger Management – Anger Management is a specific type of service which is usually informed by the practices of Cognitive Behavioural Therapy (CBT). CBT believes that a person's cognitions – defined by different theorists as beliefs/thoughts or meanings (Gipps, 2012) – negatively distort the way that individuals perceive themselves and the world around them (McLeod, 2019). Unlike Narrative Therapy, this distortion is typically understood as irrational thinking (Ellis, 1995) or cognitive deficiencies (Beck, 1987). Consequently, within CBT, a therapist's role is to offer perspective and help a service-user to manage their disruptive thoughts and behaviours. When applied to the feelings, thoughts and behaviours associated with anger management, practitioners do not attempt to remove the sensation of anger. Instead, they seek to reduce the physiological arousal and negative thinking that is thought to lead to socially unaccepted expressions or depressive symptoms. Strategies include relaxation techniques such as breathing, visualisation and calming words, which manage the depths of anger that is felt (American Psychological Association, 2022). Another strategy is cognitive restructuring, which manages the frequency that anger is experienced by challenging binary thinking and excessive swearing (APA, 2022).

Applying the Learning to Creative Health

The final consideration I will explore in this chapter is how readers might apply this frame within the context of Creative Health. To do this, I will explore some examples relating to health promotion. Health promotion involves helping members of the public to be aware of – and better understand – different health conditions and healthy lifestyles. Depending on the context of health promotion, it can be both a method for identifying relatable health experiences in the general population or a tool for improving people awareness of how they can better manage these experiences.

A great example of an informal Creative Health activity which has impacted my own life is social media content about ADHD and/or ASD. Here, a multitude of users with direct experience of ADHD and/or ASD create short reels where they act out common experiences and narrate through a neurodivergent lens. This has helped me to feel connected to others who share experiences like my own, to understand how the presentation of neurodivergence differs from medical textbook accounts, and to learn about why micro-conflicts can arise between people with neurological differences. In my own work, I have attempted to contribute to this body of online resources. However, I wanted my contribution to be less about identifying ADHD and/or ASD behaviours, and more about sharing some of the ways in which Creative Health approaches can manage difficulties associated with these neurotypes. An example of this is my blog for the National Centre for Creative Health, entitled *Creative Approaches to Health & Wellbeing: A Neurodivergent Perspective* (Hearst, 2024). The purpose of this resource is to help neurodivergent people and the people that support them (either formally or informally) to develop creative strategies for managing negative symptoms of ADHD and ASD.

Another mode of using creativity to support health promotion is via museums. A great example of this is the Everywhere and Nowhere project – 'a collaboration between the National Trust and the University of Leicester's Research Centre for Museums and Galleries that explores little known and previously untold histories of disability from across Trust sites and collections' (Research Centre for Museums and Galleries, 2023). One of the key artists in this project is Christopher Samuel, whose work 'addresses the imbalance of representation in medical and social archives to build a better understanding of the wider spectrum of the human experience' (Wellcome Collection, 2022). Christopher has been involved in a range of innovative projects over the years, which help people with disabilities to see themselves represented in art and archives, and for people without disabilities to better understand the experiences of those who do. This exemplifies the role that Creative Health can play in identifying threats to wellbeing, for those who are not necessarily experiencing the threat themselves but who have the power to help mitigate or support those who do. This reminds me of an experience I had earlier this year.

Whilst facilitating a 'huddle[1]' with people with Acquired Brain Injuries (ABIs), I came across the question of how we can improve the number of people engaging with creative outputs about ABIs. The group acknowledged that what they needed was greater awareness of their experience within the general population, yet content about their experience often wasn't engaged with until somebody acquired a brain injury or was close to somebody else who had. This, for me, points to the importance of identifying a service-providers role in identification over management. As soon as a provider prioritises this role then they can start asking these crucial design questions on how best to achieve awareness about a condition. Some of the design choices I discussed that day, looked at how to centre an audience member within the experience or narrative. For example, human libraries are a great Creative Health provision that allow members of the public to access people (rather than books) who have lived experience that they are happy to discuss and answer questions about. This personable access to information often leads to better engagement from people, compared to asking that same person to research a topic independently, as it allows the conversation to be adapted around their interests and perspectives. Alternatively, theatre productions that position health experiences within a fantastical context help audience members to feel more connected to the message which is being communicated. For example, instead of promoting a theatre production about ABIs as a story of 'other,' a marketer may choose to write a blurb which encourages the audience to consider what they would do if they suddenly lost their personality or began to fall frequently with fatigue. By inviting audiences into the experience like this, it removes the otherness of the message and encourages an awareness of ABI's as something that could happen to any of us. This heightened awareness can then lead to preventative health behaviours, better health literacy in noticing warning signs for ABI causes like stroke, and improved supportive behaviours between those with and without ABIs.

Another way that creativity can engage audiences in the identification and awareness of health conditions is through immersive simulation or re-enactment. An example of this is a short film by Elle Smart (*Impact*, 2020). In an evaluation I conducted into the use of filmmaking for therapeutic purposes (*The Lasting Benefits of Random Acts*, 2021), Elle explained that she used inconsistent editing techniques to replicate the experience of PTSD for audience members:

> I looked specifically at how post-production can influence empathy. I did studies into kinetic empathy, stuck electrodes onto people, and had them watch different types of edit to see how their muscles reacted [...] shifting the pace quite erratically, rather than it just being fast paced [...] I could see that their muscles were tensing over time and their heart was pounding [...] that makes you feel more on edge and that's PTSD. That's the hyper-arousal side of things.

It is this immersive nature of artistic experiences that can distinguish artistic forms of health promotion from traditional methods, and ultimately lead to more successful outcomes.

Final Thoughts...

Whilst the distinction between identifying and managing threats to wellbeing may be more intuitive than some of the other frames of reference in this framework, participant data suggests that there is a lack of communication about this distinction. I hope that by exploring a range of contexts in which this frame can come in useful, I have demonstrated that it is a tool for distinguishing the role of different services from one another, building trust, and providing the lens for improved collaboration. I argue that it is through this development of research and services that Creative Health advocates can provide the holistic care that many of us strive for.

Note

1 A huddle is a co-production space between health service providers and people with lived experience of mental health in relation to a particular theme or demographic. The conversation is facilitated through artistic means and aims to improve the quality of provisions available for the mental health experience being explored. Huddles are delivered through the National Centre for Creative Health, UK, and are funded by The Baring Foundation.

References

Aje (2022) Interview with Jane Hearst.

American Psychological Association (2022) *Control Anger Before It Controls You*. Available from: https://www.apa.org/topics/anger/control [Accessed 12/10/22].

Beck, A.T. (1987) Cognitive models of depression. *Journal of Cognitive Psychotherapy*, 1(1), pp. 5–37.

Denborough, D. (2014) *Retelling the Stories of Our Lives: Everyday Narrative Therapy to Draw Inspiration and Transform Experience*. 1st Edition. New York; London: W.W. Norton & Company.

Ekundayo (2021) Interview with Jane Hearst.

Ellis, A. (1995) Thinking processes involved in irrational beliefs and their disturbed consequences. *Journal of Cognitive Psychotherapy*, 9(2), pp. 105–116.

Gayle (2021) Interview with Jane Hearst.

Gipps, R.G.T. (2012) *CBT: A Philosophical Critique*. [Online] Philosophical Perspectives in Clinical Psychology. Available at: http://clinicalphilosophy.blogspot.com/2012/04/cbt-philosophical-critique.html [Accessed 01/10/2022].

Hayward, M. (2022) *Level 1 Training in Narrative Therapy*. [In-Person Training] The Institute of Narrative Therapy. 3–7 October. Available at: https://www.theint.co.uk/training/level-one/

Hearst, J. (2024) *Creative Approaches to Health & Wellbeing: A Neurodivergent Perspective*. [Online] National Centre for Creative Health: News and Blogs. Available at: https://ncch.org.uk/blog/creative-approaches-to-health-wellbeing-a-neurodivergent-perspective [Accessed 07/06/2024].

Impact. (2020) [Narrative Short] Directed by Elle Samrt. Hereford. Channel 4, Random Acts.

McLeod, S. (2019) *Cognitive Behavioral Therapy – CBT*. Available at: https://www.simplypsychology.org/cognitive-therapy.html [Accessed 17/10/2022].

Ngoen (2022) Interview with Jane Hearst.

Redstone, A. (2022) *Level 1 Training in Narrative Therapy*. [In-Person Training] The Institute of Narrative Therapy. 3–7 October. Available at: https://www.theint.co.uk/training/level-one/

Research Centre for Museums and Galleries (2023) *Everywhere and Nowhere: Exploring Histories of Disability Across the National Trust*. [Online] University of Leicester. Available at: https://le.ac.uk/rcmg/research-archive/everywhere-and-nowhere#:~:text=Abbey%20National%20Trust-,Everywhere%20and%20Nowhere%20is%20a%20collaboration%20between%20the%20National%20Trust,Accele.ation%20Account%3B%20the%20University%20of [Accessed 22/10/2024].

The Lasting Benefits of Random Acts (2021) [Documentary] Directed by *The Lasting Benefits of Random Acts.* https://www.youtube.com/watch?v=c5b6LTK6DoQ

Wellcome Collection (2022) *Wellcome Collection's Upcoming Programme, Autumn 2022 to Spring 2023.* [Online] Wellcome Collection. Available at: https://wellcomecollection.org/pages/wellcome-collection-s-upcoming-programme--autumn-2022-to-spring-2023 [Accessed 22/10/2024].

Chapter 14

Internal or External Resources

In this chapter, we'll be discussing the question: *does the researcher/service-provider support service-users to attain internal or external resources?* This question was developed in response to a critique of resilience theory which first emerged in my reading of MacKinnon and Derickson's (2013) paper on resourcefulness. Here, they distinguished between the responsibilities of an individual and the responsibilities of social institutions and policies. Aligning this with the concept of internal and external threats explored in Chapter 9, the language of internal and external resources differentiates between resilience mechanisms we hold internally and physical tools/practical support we access externally.

Defining Internal and External Resources

Internal resources describe skills, strengths, and guiding principles that heighten an individual's ability to survive through moments of increased pressure or trauma.

External resources are usually tangible or measurable assets that individuals can own or access, which reduce the number of threats that they face.

Utilising this language, we're able to develop the theory proposed by MacKinnon and Derickson's (2013) that wellbeing results from an effective negotiation of responsibility between individuals and institutions rather than a duty of one or the other. Where the language of internal and external resources brings clarity to this concept is that it defines the purpose of each type of resource. Specifically, external resources affect the *intensity* of threats that an individual is faced with, whereas internal resources determine the *threshold* of the individual to deal with these threats. Lack of wellbeing, therefore, can be the result of either threats exceeding the intensity that an individual can reasonably withstand or an individual holding a low tolerance in their response to threats. This clarity is important when considering a service-provider's role, as it allows them to accurately communicate about the share of responsibility that they deem reasonable between the individual

DOI: 10.4324/9781003423317-20

and the systems that affect them. Adding to this, the service-provider can be explicit in detailing the portion of responsibility they would like to provide and the reasoning for their chosen scope of responsibility. This makes the boundaries of a relationship clearer to the service-user and the response to new context or dynamics can be more readily predicted, informing their autonomy and decision-making.

The Unique Selling Point of the Arts

Where artistic providers choose to hold a supportive role relating to external resources, they can consider a range of modes. This can include artistic advocacy campaigns, workshops that support the accessibility of physical resources, or art materials which provide practical support. In some circumstances, the art itself can be the external resource, such as art in hospitals, which has been shown to impact the speed of patient recovery (Eminovic et al., 2021).

Based on my research, however, Creative Health services appear to primarily focus on the development of internal resources. The arts hold a strength in their ability to explore meaning within various forms of knowing and use this to develop values, power relations, strength of expression, interpersonal skills, motivation, and self-awareness. These are all vital protective factors within the development of internal resources. The ability of the arts to empower in this way is a Unique Selling Point (USP) which distinguishes them from more authoritative support systems.

The following interview excerpt provides an example of an authoritative support system to demonstrate more clearly where the arts can differentiate and what is missing from current communications about this USP.

When Kris was making changes in their life, they desired reassurance that their life had purpose. This inspired them to turn to the church. They reflected, 'When I first started going, it actually helped me loads. I felt really good [...] until they got right into my life. I was like "whoa, whoa, back off, stay away"' (Kris, 2021). In this story, the church understood itself as the source of meaning and, therefore, believed that it could dictate the shape of this meaning. It failed to recognise that meaning is generated within the individual, even when they choose to align to a religion. This was exposed in Kris's observations on their yoga practice:

> What [the church] realise, is that Yoga does teach you that you don't need anything external [...] I didn't need to do what the church was telling me to do when, actually, to heal myself and to do good by others, if I just am at peace with myself then I fix all them things anyway [...] [whereas] they wanted me to lean on all those external things.
>
> (Kris, 2021)

This example illustrated how a support service can become toxic when it fails to recognise the impact of an individual's agency and the service's role as a facilitative resource. Imposing a structure of meaning that is incongruent with an individual's internal narrative can be harmful, which is why the method of empowerment that is characteristic of many arts provisions becomes exemplary.

There are external resources – akin to the church – which do provide a sense of alignment and purpose for some individuals and communities. However, the power of internal resources is that they allow the individual to hold independence. This independent source of wellbeing is more readily controlled by an individual, which gives them the ability to make it more sustainable. Since this is where the arts thrive, they have an opportunity to promote themselves as enriching, sustainable, and non-authoritative.

Three Methods of Attaining Internal Resources

Because internal resources carry so many strengths, I present three methods of facilitating the development of internal resources. I identified these nuanced approaches via participant stories and adjacent literature:

1 Unconditional Positive Regard
2 Reference Points of Viable Possibilities
3 Facilitative Environments for Adaptation

Unconditional Positive Regard (UPR) is a concept that was created by Stanley Standal (1954) and popularised by Carl Rogers (1956) within his development of humanistic psychology. It describes a state of complete acceptance of a person, regardless of their alignment with one's own values or point of view (Jacobson and Blundell, 2016). It is about expressing care despite the fallible nature of human beings and accepting the individual for their deeper self rather than responding to surface behaviour. Wellbeing practitioners, such as therapists, utilise the concept of UPR to help their service-user to feel seen and accepted within the user-provider relationship. This has been shown to encourage service-users to practice UPR towards themselves outside of the counselling room (Jacobson and Blundell, 2016), which creates powerful changes in their behaviour, sense of self, and overall wellbeing.

Within Kris's story of the church, they demonstrated how a lack of UPR from a service-provider can tarnish a user-provider relationship. Within other interviews, participants demonstrated what the presence of UPR looks like in their daily lives. In Ekundayo's case, they shared their story of offering UPR to their children. They unveiled three significant advantages to this value system: 1) that their children intuitively know right from wrong, 2) that they know how to hold people accountable, and 3) that they carry a great deal of self-confidence. For Ekundayo, this signified a striking difference to own experience of being a child, where the lack of regard from their abusive parent left them vulnerable to manipulation and confused about where the lines of right and wrong lay (Ekundayo, 2021).

Reference Points of Viable Possibilities (**RPVP**) refers to memories, filmic depictions, or observations of others that provide an individual with a concept of what is possible from their life. This is a concept I developed in response to several storytelling participants, who identified a flourishing childhood as a key reason for their wellbeing being so stable as an adult. Within their stories participants shared that their access to happy memories provided them with a template of what was possible from their lives, which in turn motivated their choices and provided a mental safety-net for when they faced challenges on the path towards their goals.

An example of a participant who identified RPVPs in their story was Bodhi (2022). Describing some of the assets from their childhood, Bodhi stressed the value of quality education – which, in their experience, was higher in Zambia than it was in the UK. They also found that the land they could access had provided the opportunity to roam and play. Sharing a home with a second family and a wealth of animals meant that they had access to a large community of support systems and, as the youngest child, they were particularly spoilt with attention and love. Adding to this, Bodhi experienced a significant lack of discrimination – both in terms of caste and religion – and loved the sunny warm weather of Zambia (Bodhi, 2022). Here, Bodhi described how having access to a facilitative environment as a child provided them with an example of what a good life can be like. This meant that Bodhi has, since, had the opportunity to design their life with confidence, knowing that, if things go wrong, they can trace the steps back to reignite this version of their world.

Facilitative Environments for Adaptation (**FEFA**) describes safe spaces in which an individual can reflect on their self and what they need to change to achieve better wellbeing. I use this term, specifically, to denote a space that is accessed frequently enough to either become the dominant environment reflected in a person's internal world or to counteract the negative effects of a toxic dominant environment. FEFA is another concept that I developed in response to findings within participant data. It responds to the erosive effects of negative environments and the benefits that were evidenced as these environments changed. Moreover, it captures the model used by rehabilitation centres – whereby service-users are given a space of reprieve from the environments that enabled their downfall – whilst inviting service-providers to innovate past this for users with less 'acute' needs.

Within Aje's story of disability, they provided a pertinent example of how facilitative environments have a place in community care. From hospitals whose staff supported their self-worth, to a workspace they can express themselves in; Aje has had access to, and has developed, a range of empowering environments. They explained that part of their daily routine is organising the items on their desk to be straight and choosing from a collection of perfumes, as these rituals offer them a sense of control over their environment that was lost when their disability initially developed (Aje, 2022). In contrast with this story, Samawah listed a number of environments that restricted their control. For example, their home life is led by elders and their work life is dictated by discriminative organisations and visa policies. Unlike Aje, the people in Samawah's life do not adjust around their illness, expecting Samawah, instead, to overachieve and balance many different hats (Samawah, 2022). Samawah signalled that they could benefit from having access to a space where these pressures were reduced, to provide them with the mental space to work on their wellbeing.

Applying the Learning to Creative Health

To demonstrate how this frame can be used to better understand the strengths of different Creative Health services, I will provide two examples of existing provisions.

Looking firstly at internal resources, I point to Katie Watson's therapeutic writing services. Katie is one of many providers that use the power of creative writing for therapeutic purposes. What I particularly like about Katie's promotional communication of these services is that she is specific in its intended outputs. Specifically, her website notes 'Through writing, we can begin to cultivate linguistic control over the trauma and reorganise our story, in the supportive presence of like-minded peers' (Watson, 2024). The language of *linguistic control* implicitly references an internal resource, whereby an individual can regain control of their narrative and, with this, their sense of autonomy. This service is focused on the individual and their relationship with themselves, even though it can involve a peer-to-peer narrative exploration.

In our second example, I look to the Bollywood dance classes offered by Bollyqueer.

> Bollyqueer is a dance class which centres Queer and Trans people. When you walk into a Bollyqueer class, you are not assigned any label, your gender is never assumed, and you are encouraged to dance in a way that makes your heart and body feel their happiest [...] It's a way to celebrate the magic and beauty of Bollywood dance without having to sacrifice your queerness or identity. It's a family.
>
> (Jobanputraa, 2024)

In this description of Bollyqueer's services, founder, Vinay Jobanputraa, establishes a strong identity and purpose. A specific value system is demonstrated through a range of targeted shifts in Bollywood dance representation. These shifts mark a change of environment for people who have otherwise felt excluded form- or unsafe in- traditional Bollywood dance environments. By offering this environment to LGBTQIA+ attendees, Vinay provides them with an external resource. This might be considered the access to quality and well-aligned dance tutoring. For others, the value may lie in the community this creates – a community of likeminded peers. If the latter applies, then an attendee might also begin to cultivate internal resources relating to a sense of identity and belonging, either adjusting their presentation of self in other spaces or feeling stronger and more self-assured in places that are not as affirming. The service itself, however, focuses on the external resources it can provide.

Taking the framing of internal/external resources and the methods of facilitating the development of internal resources, researchers and service-providers are able to design new services and targeted programmes. Let's say, for example, a team of Creative Health practitioners wanted to develop a wellbeing retreat. We know based on the three resource-enabling methods that it would be good to include:

- a space to reflect, away from the responsibilities of home and work environments
- access to role models and peer support to improve awareness of what is possible from life
- a judgement free retreat, where attendees are embraced as the expert in their own experiences

Thinking about the way that Creative Health activities could then be used to amplify these enablers, providers have a range of options to choose from. A selection might include:

- drama workshops, which invite you to act out who you want to be, to develop your awareness of your identify and trial different versions of your future
- visual art workshops, where you will personify a 'negative' aspect of your identity, describe its form, and reconceptualise its place within your life
- nature photography workshops, where you are encouraged to notice the little details around you, and consider who you are outside of the systems of our society
- writing workshops, which provide you with the skills to communicate your values back to those you love or associate with

By using this framing to consider the value of resources, effective interventions can be quickly designed to support service-users.

Final Thoughts...

This chapter has outlined the value in distinguishing between internal and external resources, both so that it can enable better conversation about the division of responsibility for an individual's wellbeing and to improve the compatibility of services offered to the individual. Internal and external resources are distinct from the internal and external threats explored in Chapter 9. To demonstrate we can refer to the Creative Health examples. In the case of Bollyqueer, the threat might be an internal threat, like sense of belonging or self-esteem, whereas the resources that were offered are both external – dance tuition and a community of likeminded people. In the therapeutic writing workshops, individuals have likely experiences two types of threat – the external threat which caused trauma of some kind and the internal deterioration which resulted. The goal of the writing workshop is to focus on the internal threat, by developing more internal resources. When applying this framing to your own research or service design, therefore, I recommend that you consider this relationship between frames and how this might be communicated with clarity to your intended audiences – be that service-users, commissioners, or otherwise.

References

Aje (2022) Interview with Jane Hearst.

Bodhi (2022) Interview with Jane Hearst.

Ekundayo (2021) Interview with Jane Hearst.

Eminovic, S. et al. (2021) Positive effect of colors and art in patient rooms on patient recovery after total hip or knee arthroplasty: A randomized controlled trial. *Wiener klinische Wochenschrift*, [Online] Available at: https://doi.org/10.1007/s00508-021-01936-6 [Accessed 26/01/2022].

Jacobson, S. and Blundell, A. (2016) *Unconditional Positive Regard – What It Is and Why You Need It.* [Online] Harley Therapy. Available at: https://www.harleytherapy.co.uk/counselling/unconditional-positive-regard-what-it-is-and-why-you-need-it.htm [Accessed 15/05/2020].

Jobanputraa, V. (2024) *Breaking Down Gender Norms with Bollywood Dance.* [Online] Bollyqueer. Available at: https://bollyqueer.com/about-us [Accessed 08/08/2024].

Kris (2021) Interview with Jane Hearst.

MacKinnon, D. and Derickson, K.D. (2013) From resilience to resourcefulness: A critique of resilience policy and activism. *Progress in Human Geography*, 37(2), pp. 253–270.

Rogers, C.R. (1956) Clientcentered theory. *Journal of Counseling Psychology*, 3(2), pp. 115–120.

Samawah (2022) Interview with Jane Hearst.

Standal, S.W. (1954) *The Need for Positive Regard: A Contribution to Client-Centered Therapy – Proquest.* Chicago: The University of Chicago.

Watson, K. (2024) *Writing the Self: Foundation Programme.* [Online] Katie Watson Psychotherapy. Available at: https://katiewatsonpsychotherapy.co.uk/therapeutic-writing/ [Accessed 05/07/2024].

Chapter 15

Specific or Holistic Goals

In this chapter, I ask the question: *does the service-provider hold specific or holistic goals?* This is an important frame in the Creative Health Communication Framework as it addresses one of the key tensions in Creative Health promotions. That is, different stakeholders in Creative Health have different views about what type of services they want to prioritise. Some enjoy the predictability of targeted interventions and find this an easier sell to target-based health systems. Others point out the inherent benefit of engaging with the arts and how this links to so-called 'wicked' issues; those that are multifaceted, complex, and, therefore, hard to measure or compartmentalise. As you have been exploring the chapters of this book, so far, you may have found yourself answering some of the frames with the answer 'well, I do both/multiple of those things.' For people favouring a holistic approach, that may well be the correct answer to those frames but, even if that is true, it is helpful to explain this multifaceted approach to your services-users and commissioners. These frames help you to show what 'holistic' means to you, so that you are all on the same page.

One of the reasons why this frame is an important one to include is because services which carry a focus on one specific function are often prioritised by the market. This is done for several reasons. Firstly, they are easier to communicate clearly and minimise the space for misinterpretation. Secondly, because they carry a specific goal, they are easier to measure and evaluate. Thirdly, implicit in this ability to evaluate is a sense of accountability. Conversely, holistic provisions can be overly flexible and lacking in direction, meaning that they risk service-providers reporting positive results, even if these results were not the desired outcome of the service-user.

Since I recognise that a holistic approach is part of the core philosophies of many artforms, it was important for me to consider the place of this approach within the market. In my Narrative Compositional Analysis of participants orientation charts, I observed a distinction between the types of users who benefitted from services with specific functions, and those who may be better supported through holistic approaches to care. At the centre of

DOI: 10.4324/9781003423317-21

this distinction was a difference between what I label as 'simple' and 'complex' wellbeing systems. By referring to simple and complex wellbeing systems in this chapter, I demonstrate that it is possible to have clear, actionable goals within a holistic approach to care, and I establish when a holistic approach is, in fact, more appropriate than a specified service.

Simple versus Complex Wellbeing Systems

A simple wellbeing system is defined as one where each factor affecting an individual's wellbeing is associated with a dominant wellbeing orientation (see Chapters 8 and 11). This entails that the relationship between a resource and it's affect is simple. For example, loneliness might have a strong correlation to a person's sense of social orientation. In this case, an anti-loneliness group is a simple intervention that can shift the orientation of this individual towards one of togetherness and connection.

It is important to note that simple wellbeing systems can still be associated with complex lifenarratives and extreme traumas. It is not the content of these stories that make them simple, rather this language describes the relationship between resources and their affects.

A complex wellbeing system is defined as one where factors affect several wellbeing orientations. In this case, a holistic service may be the only suitable approach as these service-users require a more comprehensive type of support. For a holistic service to be labelled as such, it may offer multiple types of resources to address the range of orientations that need support. Alternatively, it may offer a single resource, but this resource is one that is equally as complex as the factor affecting wellbeing. That is, the service is one which inherently impacts multiple aspects of an individual's wellbeing.

What is useful to clarify is that there are different conceptualisations of what holistic support entails. Some holistic approaches describe a carefully prepared combination of services which collaborate to uplift the baseline of a service-users wellbeing. Other holistic services, such as talking therapies, help a service-user to explore various aspects of their wellbeing experience but the success of these services depends on a service-user's access to other resources. In this latter scenario, the task is not to provide other resources, where there was once an absence, but instead develop the internal resources that allows a service-user to maximise the benefit of their external resources.

In the following four sections of this chapter, I will refer to stories from participant interviews to explore the differences between simple/complex wellbeing systems and their link to focused/holistic care. Through these stories I intend to show the importance of considering whether a service should be focused or holistic, particularly as it pertains to the compatibility with a service-user.

The Link between Dominating Wellbeing Factors and Focused Care

Jiva is an extroverted character with a love of social interaction and a desire to help others, yet, when they were asked to describe their wellbeing, Jiva identified a narrative of 'Me vs Us,' describing the social as dangerous and the self as the best leader for their wellbeing (Jiva, 2022). When presenting their story of wellbeing, Jiva filed all of their wellbeing factors, exclusively, into two orientations: Social Influences and Mindset. The motivation for Jiva's narrative, they explained, was their history of addictive behaviours and the circumstances in which they struggled the most. When Jiva has been swayed by the influence of others, they were more likely to drink or take drugs and become addicted to these substances. When they were focusing on their health and their goals, their positive mindset was enough to get them back on track for significant portions of time, until another social scenario affected their progress (Jiva, 2022).

What is interesting about Jiva's experience is that their lifestyle is not absent from activities which support the unaddressed orientations within their chart (as shown through their Tree of Life diagram and the accompanying commentary). For example, as somebody with a passion for their sport, the physical body has an important place in Jiva's daily activities. Moreover, they have access to compatible environments, full of people who share their hobbies. For this reason, there is a distinction between the 'active' resources they described in their coded data and the 'inactive' resources that came up in their wider discussion of self.

I use the term **active resources** to describe those that a service-user is aware of, and which are sewn into their wellbeing narratives. These may not be the only resources that affect their wellbeing, but they are the resources that feel most pertinent or obvious within their understanding of self.

Inactive resources, therefore, describe assets which have not been identified within a service-users key life narrative. On some occasions, these resources may be taken for granted because of their high levels of stability. In other scenarios, these resources may have less significant impacts or are seen to remain neutral between a service-user's experience of wellbeing at their best and worst.

This example demonstrates how wellbeing factors – or in this case narrative plot points – can be shaped by a person's perception of their life. The fact that Jiva was not experiencing an absence of resources in other orientations indicates that the social and psychological orientations are where they experience the most instability, unpredictability and/or lack of control. For this reason, the type of service Jiva could most benefit from is one where they can improve the external resources in their social orientation (i.e., friends and associates which are more supportive of Jiva's goals and compatible to their preferred lifestyle) or the internal resources connected to their psychological orientation (e.g., an enduring sense of discipline, self-control over health promoting behaviours, etc.). These are specific goals that link nicely to a simple wellbeing narrative with dominant wellbeing factors.

The Link between Rippling Disorientation, Focused Care, and Holistic Outcomes

The next example demonstrates how service-providers can become clear why it may be necessary to focus a lot of attention on one function rather than a little attention on multiple functions. This is done by acknowledging the weighted dependence of factors within a simple wellbeing system.

When Lou described their highest and lowest wellbeing stories, they identified ten different wellbeing factors. Many of these factors derived from normative social roles, such as being family oriented and having a long-term career, encountering traditional structures such as the church, and managing common struggles with money-management (Lou, 2021). Within Lou's stories they identified wellbeing factors that had both positive and negative impacts based on their context. Namely, when Lou's workplace was heavily influenced by the camaraderie they shared with their workmates it was a joyful aspect of their identity. Moreover, as a proud partner and parent, Lou's family provides them with a comforting awareness of what their role is. This combination of work and home have provided an implicit sense of meaning. Yet, when money problems disrupted this balance, and tensions began to rise in these character-defining aspects of their life, Lou became explicitly disconnected to their sense of purpose; so much so, that one New Year's Day, they stood at the side of train tracks wondering whether to take their own life (Lou, 2021).

In Lou's stories, factors connected to their family featured within multiple wellbeing orientations. Specifically, their marriage provides them with a sense of their role, which affects their psychological orientation. The birth of their children marked both joyous but physically straining moments of their life, featuring in the physiological orientation. Moreover, their children and grandchildren facilitate a large amount of social interaction, which places them into social orientation. All three of these aspects are closely interconnected, so when Lou started to feel like they were failing their partner, all three categories of wellbeing became disorientated. In this scenario, it was a psychological disorientation which put the other orientations at risk.

From Lou's interview commentary, it's possible to discern that once this psychological orientation was re-established, so too did the other aspects of their life begin to mend. Consequently, Lou's experience demonstrates that, in certain scenarios, services which support a specific orientation can have holistic benefits. This challenges the notion that specific and holistic forms of care are always distinct from one another, which supports my argument that service-providers benefit from defining what holistic means to them and validating their claims through a coherent strategy of care delivery.

I suggest that service-providers who intend to deliver a service which has a comparable relationship between a dominant orientation and its interdependent orientations should communicate the power of this ripple effect to their users. Not all service-users will be aware of the benefits of this approach without guiding language or examples from others, yet those very benefits can be tremendous. By indicating these ripple benefits, service-providers offer their users motivation to embark on a journey to wellbeing. This is important, as without this motivation the journey can feel overwhelming, and the strength of the benefits can be unclear.

Character Models versus Guiding Principles

To build on the findings from Lou's interrelated wellbeing orientations, I turn to an example from Kris's interview. Kris also created a simple wellbeing chart, yet their narrative was far more complex. By exploring their experience, this example shows how individuals can make sense of their wellbeing thanks to guiding principles, thematically compartmentalise their wellbeing stories, and shift the type of care they prefer.

Like Jiva, Kris centred their wellbeing narrative around a negotiation between the self and the external. They categorised leaning on the external as a negative thing and leaning on the internal as a positive (Kris, 2021). Yet Kris's Seven Orientations chart indicated that their narrative was much more complex in its function. Namely, rather than a conflict between social and psychological orientation, the centre of Kris's story focused on the category of spiritual orientation. Kris's relationship with factors within this category is to treat them as guiding principles rather than descriptions of character. Consequently, these guiding principles were able to penetrate surrounding orientations and influence the factors within them.

Explicitly, when Kris used to focus on other people as their guide, Kris became aware of how under-appreciated they were at their job, how countercultural they were in their actions and, consequently, how unsuited they were to their living environment. Whereas, when Kris decided to centre their choices around a narrative of self-love, they began to choose the people they allowed into their environment based on their compatibility, learnt to say no to actions that did not align to their needs, cultivated a work environment where they had freedom over their time, and chose to design conscious self-care practices. This change in narrative was supported by an attention to growth mindset which affected their view of things such as money – shifting their view away from a narrative of chasing towards it to a narrative of acceptance and awareness of fundamental needs (Kris, 2021).

What Kris's story highlights is that strength can be derived from using factors as guiding principles rather than descriptors of character, as this provides more space for adaptation. Kris developed their guiding principle to help them to compartmentalise externally focused threats, saying that everything comes down to the absence or presence of self-love, and explained that harmful actions of others are usually a reflection of their lack of self-love rather than a targeted attack. The sophistication of this narrative style and reasoning clearly demonstrated itself as a protective factor.

For service-providers who seek to offer holistic outcomes from specific interventions, they may wish to consider incorporating the logic of guiding principles into their work. Here, **Guiding Principles** describe a type of logic that can adjust to different contexts and fluctuating access to external resources. They are distinct from **Character Models** where an individual seeks to fulfil a particular social function in a particular ideal manner. The core difference is that guiding principles are more adaptable to change and less likely to deteriorate during moments of emotional strain. This means that an individual becomes protected against damaging existential crisis', maintaining a strong and autonomous sense of self and purpose. Creative Health services can support the development of guiding principles - a specific goal with holistic impacts.

The Link between Complex Wellbeing Systems and Holistic Care

To build on these examples of simple wellbeing systems, I turn to a final participant story – this one exploring a complex wellbeing system.

In Aje's interview, they went into detail about the complexity of their wellbeing and provided an exhaustive list of factors (Aje, 2022). This gave me a brilliantly clear insight into how they have nurtured the growth of positive resources within their life. Prominently, Aje's resources were evenly distributed; for almost every negative factor, they experienced in their lowest wellbeing they cultivated a positive factor in their current wellbeing system. This gives an indication that the more complex an individual's internal battle during negative times, the more complex their support systems may need to be to provide positive wellbeing.

Implicit within Aje's conceptualisation of their wellbeing is that there is not a dominant orientation associated with any of their wellbeing factors. Whilst the orientation framework offered them a method of describing the multiple ways that their wellbeing experienced disorientation during their worst wellbeing, none of these examples of disorientation were more heavily weighted than others. In cases like this, where a dominant orientation does not exist, there is little scope for a service-provider to offer a method of care which focuses on a specific type of disorientation. A holistic approach, on the other hand, can match the complexity of the service-users experience with a comprehensive form of support. Since the comprehensive nature of this support may not be implicit within the title of 'holistic' care, service-providers benefit from detailing some of the complexities of their provision. To demonstrate, I conclude this chapter with examples from the field of Creative Health.

Applying the Learning to Creative Health

To demonstrate the difference between services that hold specific or holistic goals, I will first refer to two Creative Health providers who both use the same artistic medium but to different effect.

Firstly, there is *Dance to Health*, a falls prevention programme offered by Aesop. This programme integrates physiotherapy into dance classes, with the aim of reducing hospital admissions for fall related injuries. On their website (Dance to Health, 2024), they demonstrate the need for their service with precise statistics, including '1 in 3 people aged over 65 fall each year' and 'the total annual UK cost of frailty fractures is estimated at [over] £4.4billion.' They then provide clear indication as to how their service aligns to this specific issue; 'Dance to Health reduces falls by 58%' (Aesop, 2020). This service is not without additional benefits – for example, the fun element of dance is what helps more elderly to engage with Dance to Health services than traditional prevention services in the NHS, and there is a correlation between the risk of frailty and social isolation, so the active engagement with Dance to Health can also affect wellbeing and life expectancy. However, by focusing in on a specific primary goal, Dance to Health is able to separate itself from the rest of the Creative Health market, positioning their service as a specialist in this area. They have engaged in rigorous evidence-collecting to show how their service affects their core aims, which aligns well with the evidence-concerned health systems of the UK.

Comparing to this is *Move Dance Feel*, a cancer supporting dance service for women who had or have cancer, or who are caring for somebody who has cancer. Like Dance to Health, Move Dance Feel has a clear understanding of its identity in the healthcare market, in that it specialises in cancer support and has a target audience of women. However, Move Dance Feel is distinct from Dance to Health as it approaches cancer care from a holistic lens. This means that service-users are invited into the space, bringing with them unique stories and emotional responses to their situation, and the dance service supports them where they are at. It does not aim to reduce their risk of cancer – though there is some indicative evidence to suggest that engagement with movement reduces the risk of some cancers, such as breast cancer (Boardman et al., 2023) – instead focusing on the wellbeing of its attendees. The texture and expression of this wellbeing differs from person to person, but that does not mean that Move Dance Feel is without evidence of its own. A partnered research project (Wakeling and Jenkins, 2019; The National Centre for Creative Health, 2023) found that benefits for participants included:

- greater joy
- improved sleep
- improved memory
- increased confidence

- enhanced cognitive performance
- increased sense of body appreciation
- reduced feelings of depression, worry and fear
- enhanced energy and a reduction in feelings of fatigue
- enhanced strength, balance, coordination, and range of motion
- enhanced sense of creativity and imaginative thinking
- enhanced sense of connection to others
- increased sense of safety and support
- reduced feelings of loneliness
- increased concentration
- improved stamina
- improved mood

What this type of evidence demonstrates is that Move Dance Feel offer a service which compliments clinical cancer services, rather than replacing them. It helps individuals with cancer, and their support network, to experience the difficulties of their journey in a more gentle and supported way, with more moments of joy and reprieve. They are able to feel better connected to others, reducing their risk of long-term mental and physical health complications, beyond the cancer journey. Initially, this may position them in the third sector, reducing their likelihood of attaining commissioning from clinical health pots. However, as we see greater movement towards Integrated Care Systems, considerations of 'wicked' issues, and a culture of person-centred, preventative care, we can hope to see greater funding towards this type of service in the future from public health and ICB integrated funding streams. It is also the type of service that is increasingly being prioritised by arts and heritage funders, who are keen to see wellbeing benefits for participants of the services they support.

With these two examples in mind, I would like to turn to one final case study. Here, I want to demonstrate what a service might look like when it sits between focused and holistic care. Specifically, this example demonstrates what a service can look like when it has specific but multiple intended outcomes.

In Shropshire, Telford and Wrekin ICS region, in the UK, healthcare providers identified an issue with Children and Young People's (CYP) management of asthma. One of the issues which prevented CYP from appropriately using their inhalers and engaging in other health-promoting behaviours was the stigma associated with their asthma and their care needs. This exacerbated issues, causing CYP to access health services that could have been avoided. A healthcare partnership considering this issue involved the Integrated Care Board, which is concerned with clinical outcomes, the public health team, which focuses on prevention and childhood development, and community partners, who supported the collective mission to provide more personalised care. Creative Health was identified as a potential solution and was trialled locally with a group of CYP. Here, poetry and singing were used to increased lung health without the stigma of traditional methods. The pilot was a great success as it not only improved lung health (the clinical outcome), but also improved CYP engagement with positive asthma related behaviours and services, and demonstrated significant benefits for speech development. This pilot is now used to promote the use of poetry and singing for CYP asthma and has encouraged health providers to consider where Creative Health may be able to support other CYP health priorities. The success of this initiative relied on a cross-sector partnership; something which is often an important enabler for Creative Health commissioning. This shows, therefore, the benefits of taking a specific yet multiple-outcome approach to service outcomes, as each partner was able to align one of the benefits to their own disparate agendas, whilst working in a collaborative manner. The future of integrated care will depend on these types of partnerships, and it is through this approach that we can move towards a more comprehensive form of healthcare.

Final Thoughts...

Throughout this chapter, I have attempted to demonstrate the importance of distinguishing between specific and holistic services. This serves two key functions. Firstly, by considering the nature of specific or holistic services as they pertain to service-users, researchers and service-providers are better able to articulate the compatibility of their approach to different ways of thinking and targeted wellbeing needs. Secondly, the communication of outputs affects the way that a service is placed within the marketplace. Creative Health advocates who wish to receive funding for their work are able to use this frame to identify appropriate commissioning partners and understand how their service or promotional communication may need to adapt in order to connect to partners from different disciplinary backgrounds. Moreover, those who are interested in shifting the cultures of healthcare in the future can use this frame to consider the relationship between specific and holistic approaches to care, as they relate to Integrated Care Systems and personalisation, and use this to their advantage when discussing their vision for growth. This framing supports the pragmatic implementation of systems change, developing the type of healthcare landscape that many creatives crave for, whilst acknowledging, respecting, and responding to the practical benefits that cause targeted interventions to be prioritised at present.

References

Aesop (2020) *Dance to Health. Phase 1 Roll-out 'test and learn' Evaluation Report.* Oxfordshire: Aesop.

Aje (2022) Interview with Jane Hearst.

Boardman, R. et al. (2023) *Social Value of Movement and Dance*. London: Sport + Recreation Alliance.

Dance to Health (2024) *Our Impact*. [Online] Dance to Health. Available at: https://dancetohealth.org/about-us/our-impact/ [Accessed 04/09/2024].

Jiva (2022) Interview with Jane Hearst.

Kris (2021) Interview with Jane Hearst.

Lou (2021) Interview with Jane Hearst.

The National Centre for Creative Health (2023) *Move Dance Feel Case Study*. [Online] Case Studies. Available at: https://ncch.org.uk/case-studies/move-dance-feel [Accessed 13/07/2024].

Wakeling, K. and Jenkins, E. (2019) *A Service Evaluation of Move Dance Feel: A Dance Project for Women Living With or Beyond Cancer*. London: Move Dance Feel.

Chapter 16

Resilience Strategies

This chapter explores the final frame of section two in the Creative Health Communication Framework, which looks at what the role of the service-provider is in supporting against a threat to wellbeing. The frame asks: *is the service-provider informed by a particular resilience strategy?*

Earlier in this book, in Chapter 6, I explained how the language of resilience aligns well with the marketplace, as it discusses wellbeing in terms of accumulation of emotional wealth, the maintenance of emotionally supportive assets, and the trade of protective resources. This onus of the individual aligns with the philosophy of free-market capitalism, in which a person is self-made. Moreover, the language of resilience is integrated into our common language, meaning that both healthcare professionals and members of the public are both familiar with its usage. In Chapter 8, I evaluated whether this was suitable language to incorporate into the Creative Health Communication Framework, considering the effects this would have on the wellbeing of our target audiences.

In this chapter, I will reflect on the nuances of the four primary terms taken from resilience theory and will use participant stories to explore the pros and cons of this language. Once the terms have been explored for their safe and appropriate usage, I will follow each story with an example of how this resilience technique has appeared in a Creative Health activity or approach. Through this, I hope to demonstrate how we can make better use of language which already penetrates into common usage in our society. As with many of the other frames, this will help researchers and service-providers to ensure that the resilience they refer to in their communication matches the understanding held by those that they are communicating with.

Resiliency

Traditionally, the term **resiliency** is used to describe a system or individual's ability to bounce back following a stressor. Coming originally from the field of engineering, resiliency assumes a single optimum state – in this case, it

DOI: 10.4324/9781003423317-22

would be a single optimum way of being well or attaining wellbeing. In my version of resiliency, I consider the relationship between stability and the base-line of wellbeing. If an individual's wellbeing has a low baseline, then the return to this state may not be enough to be deemed good wellbeing. Likewise, just because a person's wellbeing is stable – and thus, holds high resiliency – does not mean that the state of their wellbeing is in a high enough state of joy and fulfilment. In this version of resiliency, some instability, coupled with a higher baseline of wellbeing, may actually be better for the individual than stability alone. This accounts for the evolving state of individuals, their social contexts, life events, life narratives, and guiding principles. States of transition can be beneficial if they are leading to higher baseline wellbeing, via stronger guiding principles and more compatible environments and resources.

This nuance is necessary to avoid the sometime reductive application of resiliency within wellbeing support. However, there is still a place for bouncing back, within particular contexts and with service-users who resonate with this goal. The evidence from participant interviews suggests that a strategy of resiliency is best used when supporting a service-user with short-term emotional distress. The objective, in this case, is to prevent these negative emotions from turning into a perpetual state of negative wellbeing. This might be particularly useful during periods of increased stress, such as short-term hospitalisation for a physical health concern. Other uses may be applied to a service-users daily use of emotional intelligence.

Examples of participants who commented on the act of resiliency were Winnie and Gayle. Winnie said, 'If something bad happened I try not to remember it [...] I mean there always are down things – things that make you sad, things that make you cross – but there's no point in staying cross' (Winnie, 2022). Meanwhile Gayle maintained,

> I think in life you face every day, what happens to you, and then you forget it, move on, don't you [...] you've just got to say a little prayer and get on with it because it's only you that can do it.
>
> (Gayle, 2021)

Importantly, even participants like these, who favour resiliency, held ideas of when it was no longer an appropriate strategy. To demonstrate, I turn to Gayle's experience of bereavement.

Gayle expressed that they've had a rich life, full of joyful experiences and favourable value systems. They indicated that their baseline of wellbeing had been high throughout their lifetime, even though they have lived through great highs and lows emotionally speaking:

> I sit at night, and I think 'I've had a very, very good life... A really, really, very good life' [...] I've had many ups and downs and the pains and the

> cries [...] I've had a lot of sorrow. I've had sorrow like everybody else. I've had heartbreak. But on the whole I have had a good life.
>
> (Gayle, 2021)

Gayle appeared to value the dynamic nature of their emotional experience holding it as distinct from their stable wellbeing. Gayle then described their worst memory – that of their partner dying:

> I found [them] and bless [them]... [They] laid there and it was ever so cold. [They were] shivering. The nurses were with [them] and I said, '[they're] ever so cold'. So, [the nurse] said '[your partner's] been waiting for you'. And I just held [my partner's] hand and touched [their] head [...] And [they] just looked at me and smiled... and [they] died just like that. It was terrible. I wouldn't wish that on anybody. And I thought it was absolutely dreadful.
>
> (Gayle, 2021)

In this context, the strategy of resiliency was no longer appropriate. They had lost their greatest support system, a source of joy, and a means of companionship; all significant resources that affect the shape of their wellbeing. But to treat this only as a narrative of resilience, where resources can be substituted and negotiated, ignores the fact that they lost much more than this on that day. They loved their partner, despite their partner's ability to provide Gayle with wellbeing resources or not. Gayle felt great pain, not because of their inability to survive without their partner, but because they wholeheartedly did not want to.

Through this, I demonstrate, both, that the give-and-take language of the marketplace can be entirely inappropriate in certain discussions of wellbeing, and that the logic of resiliency fails to account for moments – like that of grief – where an individual may want to acknowledge and feel the loss of a 'resource' *despite* it resulting in a dip in their emotional state of mind. In scenarios like these, the language of 'bouncing back' is inapt, as the individual often does not want to return to the same state that they were in previously, if they cannot share that space with something or someone they hold dear. A better option, in this case, may be to re-member[1] their stories with the person and foster a new relationship with the values that person contributed to their life. This narrative therapy technique allows for the presence of these memories and values to remain stitched into the core of an individual's life narrative, creating a new and evolving type of wellbeing that is still rich with meaning.

Resiliency in the Context of Creative Health

Creative Health Champion, Melanie Thompson, is a GP, a Co-Clinical Director of Southeast Telford Primary Care Network, and is part of the

Shropshire, Telford and Wrekin Health and Wellbeing Board. Melanie has a passion for promoting mental wellbeing, both for her patients and the healthcare workforce. One way that she promotes creativity in health is by referencing the different chemical states of the brain and how they affect both our emotional state and on-going health. These three states were originally proposed by Paul Gilbert (2009), Professor of Clinical Psychology at University of Derby and founder of The Compassionate Mind Foundation. They are labelled 'Drive and Excitement,' 'Threat and Protection,' and 'Contentment, Soothing and Social Safety' (Gilbert, 2009).

In a state of Drive and Excitement, a person feels alert and engaged, working from a place of hopefulness and ambition. The primary chemical causing this state is dopamine, with other positive feeling chemicals being present such as oxytocin, serotonin and endorphins. In a work context, this state can often be the initial driver of highly productive people. However, when work capacity is stretched or deadlines mount up - as is often experienced in modern healthcare contexts - the threat system is activated. Threat and Protection is fuelled by adrenaline and cortisol, two chemicals which fuel the continuation of high productivity via negative emotional expressions such as anxiety, shame, and anger. Melanie explains that many GP's attempt to flick between these two states, to maintain their standards of delivery, but without access to the third state they risk reducing the quality of their work outputs.

In a state of Contentment, Soothing, and Social Safety, the body is encouraged to rest. This rest is necessary for the production of sufficient opiates and oxytocin to maintain wellbeing and prepare the mind for greater creativity. For people who regularly disregard time to rest, they will experience a decline in their ability to problem solve, recall memories, bond with others, or communicate in a caring manner. This showcases the vital link between rest and creativity, and demonstrates its place within a person's ability to 'bounce back.' In this case, a healthy movement between emotional states is what provides an individual with a sense of overall emotional equilibrium and stability in wellbeing.

Resistance

Resistance is another measurement tool that derives from Engineering (Angeler and Allen, 2016). It describes the ability of a system to withstand outside pressures without changing its core state. If we interpret this within the field of wellbeing, then it describes a person who can keep pushing through, despite pressures on their wellbeing. A clear example of where resistance was discussed within the participant interviews was when people experienced work-related stress. In these scenarios, many participants described their attempts to compartmentalise the pressures of their work to make them more manageable and resist the impact to their health. Other instances of resistance, which emerged during participant interviews, were in reaction to social vulnerabilities or misjustices. Jiva, for example, holds a strong conviction that they have 'no time for negativity' (Jiva, 2022). This can be seen as an example of resistance, as they pre-emptively choose to resist negative forces. Through Jiva's storytelling they showed that they do not experience a life that lacks negative experiences, but rather their attempt to resist internalising this negativity protects them from allowing it to become part of the lens in which they read the world.

Within my critique of resistance, I identified the dangers of **over-resistance**. Over-resistance describes acts of resistance which prevent an individual from accessing love and support, or from releasing negative emotions that are trapped within them. A pertinent example came from Ekundayo. Ekundayo explained a lesson that they and their siblings had taught one another; to 'be resilient, confident and just powerful in everything and... even when you're not, you fake it' (Ekundayo, 2021). They explained that whilst this strategy helped them to survive through childhood abuse, it also prevented others from spotting the signs that this abuse was occurring. Moreover, I noted that there were limits to the protective nature of resistance in Ekudayo's story – evidenced by all of Ekundayo's siblings self-harming and Ekundayo being hospitalised after a suicide attempt (Ekundayo, 2021). Ekundayo also expressed that they had got so used to resisting the negative effects of abuse, that they failed to set standards of behaviour for others – such as Ekundayo's ex-partner who also became abusive (Ekundayo, 2021). This story suggests that resisting, albeit necessarily within toxic environments, can encourage an individual to fake strength despite the environment, stunting their ability to consider and develop boundaries once the toxicity has been escaped from.

Resistance in the Context of Creative Health

Whilst a strategy of resistance can be one which lacks the sophistication to facilitate meaningful change in many individual contexts, it does hold an important place in the response to group/societal injustices. These injustices are slow to change, necessitating perseverance in the pursuit of social change. Creative Health research and services, therefore, can be particularly impactful in the space of artistic activism. Artistic activism brings together members of a community and their allies, to cathartically express their experience of injustices and creatively reimagine what a better future might entail.

Creative media can also be used to signal a step change in this vision of progress, responding to inequalities of various kinds. One such example, coming from my own work, is a children's book entitled *Aspire To* (Hearst, 2021). *Aspire To* was created in response to research by Aaron Toogood (De Montfort University, 2020), which found that a child's postcode affects their career aspirations, with children from poorer neighbourhoods conceptualising 'out of reach' jobs from as young as 10. Toogood proposed that this was an issue with representation and role models, so I investigated the university subjects which had issues with diverse representation. Once the most under-represented community-subject relationships were identified, I researched into staff, students and alumni from De Montfort University – where I was studying at the time – to see who fit these characteristics. Fourteen people were selected to then appear in a children's book, with a two-page spread per person sharing their story. This book functioned to resist and counteract the narrative that these demographics do not belong in these types of roles. The books were distributed to schools and libraries across the city, receiving positive feedback from the targeted demographics. I hoped it would contribute towards greater aspirations from children in Leicester.

In this example of resistance there were two key stakeholders. Firstly, was my role as lead creative. I belong to a number of disadvantaged/minoritised demographics, including working class, LGBTQIA+, and neurodivergent. This has given me some insights into career barriers. However, I do not belong to any of the groups who were experiencing the most disadvantage related to their preferred career aspiration. This insider–outsider status allowed me to remain emotionally strong, whilst serving a social change agenda that would benefit others. This is one type of resistance which is important to consider in the space of Creative Health. In addition, were the people who contributed to the book and the families who accessed this literary resource. Using the book as inspiration, these people have the opportunity to resist with greater ease, as they now have access to an alternative story – one of hope and possibility. Importantly, this application of resistance relies on a giving relationship between the research/service-provider and the beneficiary of their work.

Adaptive Capacity

Adaptive Capacity is a measurement tool originating from the field of Ecological Resilience, which describes the ability of a system to maintain a positive state of one form or another by adjusting during moments of change (Angeler and Allen, 2016). Contextualising this concept within the field of wellbeing, I propose that adaptive capacity is best understood as the adaptability of an individual when faced with unexpected hurdles or their ability to engage with periods of destabilisation during journeys of self-development. An interesting example of this type of adaptation came from Kris's interview.

When Kris was a child, they experienced sexual abuse from one of their parents. In their adulthood, they had to learn how to adapt their reaction to different kinds of external stimuli so that they could not only overcome the negative impacts of this abuse but actively grow (Kris, 2021). Below is their description of one such scenario, where they mindfully sought to overcome an automatic trauma response.

> I remember when [my partner] first moved in with me. And [they] came home from work, in their blue overalls, and [they] came to just come give

> me a kiss. And at first I was like, 'whoaaaa'. [...] and straightaway in that moment, I was like, 'What's my whoa about?', 'Why have I just leaned away?'. And it all happened in a split second. And I realised that my [abusive parent] used to pick me up from school in blue overalls. [...] And I was like, 'I just need to make a new memory out of this' [...] I don't want it to affect [my partner] or to affect us. And [they were] like, 'are you okay?!' and I was like 'yeah, yeah, kiss me, kiss me... We need to do this. It's healthy and I have to get through it; it doesn't matter how grossed out I feel, I got to do it'.
>
> (Kris, 2021)

Explicit in this story was the desire for change and the active responsibility to make change happen, despite moments of discomfort. Throughout Kris's stories, they showcased a willingness to experiment, be wrong, embrace chaos, and discover unexpected solutions. These qualities are important components of life narrative adaptation. But whilst this may be one of the strongest forms of adaptive capacity, it is not the only way of conceptualising it.

In one form of adaptive capacity, a person begins in a state where they are suffering with internal deterioration (see Chapter 9). Upon exposure to a new, healthier form of love their entire wellbeing system is reshaped. This reflects the experience of Ekundayo, whose children inspired a new sense of hope and purpose. This sense of purpose was enough to motivate Ekundayo to make significant changes in their life and become more than a survivor of childhood abuse (Ekundayo, 2021).

In another form of adaptive capacity, a person begins in a neutral state. They experience an external threat (see Chapter 9) and choose to cultivate a sense of love and purpose as a defence against this threat. This was true in Bodhi's relationship with work, whereby workplace stress was an external threat to wellbeing, but their desire to love and support their family proved strong enough to counteract this threat (Bodhi, 2022).

A third type of adaptive capacity involves a person who is brought up in an environment that provided them with internal resources (see Chapter 14). At the time that they were given these resources, they did not yet have a purpose for them. But, when they were presented with an external threat further on in life, the individual had the reserves ready to respond to this fight. In Devan's experience of overcoming depression, they described this type of discovery of unused internal resources that were available thanks to the lessons they learnt from one of their parents when they were a child (Devan, 2021).

A final example of adaptive capacity involves a person who decides to prearm themselves against predictable threats to wellbeing. By the time that the threat has arrived the individual is already prepared and is not impacted by the pressures this threat develops. Thanks to this, they make it out of the other side in a neutral state. An example of where this has featured in participant interviews is in Gayle's experience with societal poverty. They said, 'like everybody else in that [...] generation, [we] used to keep a list of what rent, groceries, you know...' (Gayle, 2021).

What these examples demonstrate is that individuals have different ways of negotiating resources and values. One way that researchers and service-providers can better apply a strategy of adaptive capacity in their work with service-users is by discussing it alongside Adaptive Choice. Where adaptive capacity describes the ability to change, **adaptive choice** recognises a person's motivation to enact this change. A researcher's or service-provider's role can either be to increase a service-user's *capacity* by reducing the barriers that are created by different systems or they can help a service-user to explore their values and determine what is their most beneficial *choice*.

Adaptive Capacity in the Context of Creative Health

The creative arts can have great impact on strengthening an individual's adaptive capacity, particularly when helping people to model alternative realities. This might include provisions such as journaling, mood board creation, drama exercises, filmmaking, and bibliotherapy. An example of where I have made use of this type of re-imagining activity is via Role-Playing Games (RPGs) like Dungeons and Dragons (D&D).

Within my first D&D campaign, I played a character called Elowyn. Elowyn was a character obsessed with discovering animals and investigating the properties of nature. Within her communication with other characters, I had to consider what her motivations may be. Often, they were linked to information gathering. Where this information was not available, I often concluded that there was no motivation, therefore, she may not stay in the conversation. This could lead to her being abrupt in her social disconnection or intolerant of small talk. Elsewhere in the campaign, the emotional response of Elowyn surprised other players. They viewed her as a chaotic character, yet I could see clearly how her motivations shaped every interaction. As the game progressed, I started to recognise that Elowyn was a symbol of my own neurodivergence. She *acted* in ways that I *thought*. This made me more aware of how and why I masked in my real life. As I continued to explore how Elowyn developed as a character or how other players interpreted her presence in the campaign, I learnt more about who I could become and how I wanted to relate to my neurodiversity. It was a cathartic, engaging and gentle way of exploring a complex experience – one full of diverse emotional experiences and equally complex modelling.

This access to relatable but fictional lived experience allowed me to strengthen my adaptive capacity, developing more sophisticated boundaries, principles, and sense of self. It is experiences like this that epitomise the strengths of Creative Health and set the discipline apart from other health and wellbeing provisions. Supporting adaptive capacity can be a preventative measure, supporting people against specific obstacles whilst also teaching them beneficial ways of thinking during future challenges.

Functional Diversity

Functional diversity is a term used to describe the value of different components within a system – in this case a wellbeing system – and their overall impact. Here, components that provide multiple functions are particularly facilitative during moments of change. Consequently, the measurement of functional diversity acknowledges the relative importance of different components on the systems survival. Within the field of wellbeing, I propose that functional diversity represents the power of a single resource to provide multiple benefits to a service-user, where another resource provides only one.

In Ngoen's (2022) interview they were able to identify a wide range of factors that affected their wellbeing – both positive and negative. Some of these wellbeing factors held a single impact whilst others were closely linked to factors identified elsewhere in their story. For example, when categorising factors into the seven orientations activity (see Chapter 8), Ngoen identified that when they were around toxic people it affected both the quality of their external environment (environmental orientation) as well as their internal mindset (psychological orientation). Similarly, unjust work practices not only affected their time (temporal orientation) but also their sense of justice and order (ability to orientate). Elsewhere, factors were connected more loosely, such as hazardous wires on the roads and green spaces (both of which were filed under environmental orientation), convenient and good transportation (temporal orientation), and their ultimate link back to basic minimum living conditions (ability to orientate).

This example demonstrates how the way that a service-user makes sense of different wellbeing factors impacts the functional diversity of each factor and the type of response that a researcher or service provider may be able to offer them. In Ngoen's story, for example, they made a link between their high school experience and a lack of critical thinking (Ngoen, 2022). Whilst Ngoen could not escape the need to go through education, a service-provider could have delivered critical thinking workshops within their school to improve the quality of this environment. This illustrates that the more developed a description of threat or resource is, the more that innovation can occur, and opportunities can be created.

Elsewhere, a way that service-providers can help users with more simple descriptions of their experience is to investigate the functional diversity of their stories and make space for this innovation.

Functional Diversity in the Context of Creative Health

In my final example of applying these principles to the field of Creative Health, I want readers to consider not only how they can support service-users via these concepts but also how they can be used to support their own enterprise. The field of Creative Health is one that is full of all the tensions you might expect when bridging two disparate industries – culture and healthcare. Funding, in this context, can be unpredictable and highly volatile, necessitating resilience in order to survive as a business or area of research specialism. In this case, the rationale of functional diversity aligns well with the concept of diversification of services.

The diversification of services involves an enterprise expanding the types of services they can offer under different circumstances. When resources are limited, the best diversification strategy should not involve the attainment of new non-financial resources – such as equipment, buildings, staff, or skillsets. Rather, this strategy asks service-providers to consider how they can use their existing resources to offer something new, by shifting the assembly of resources in their offer. For example, when I worked as a freelance filmmaker, my skills were in writing compelling stories, facilitating meaningful interviews, creating quality video outputs, safeguarding wellbeing, understanding the entrepreneurial landscape, and promoting social good. My ideal service was a therapeutic filmmaking service, which involved participatory engagement from members of the public who would create short-form narrative films. However, as I learnt to diversify my offering, I found myself giving guest lectures on developing a film business, creating marketing films for social change organisations, conducting interviews for book content or research, delivering motivational talks about my experience of wellbeing, and supporting businesses in their promotional pitches. None of these new services required me to learn new skills or invest in new equipment, saving me valuable time and energy. By diversifying in this way, I could survive the early stages of a freelance career without sacrificing my financial security.

This same concept can be applied to stories of wellbeing. Much like the entrepreneurial scene, the goal of maintaining wellbeing can sometimes feel like a difficult balancing act. By helping research participants or service-users to consider what they *do* have access to and how these skills/resources can be applied in new ways, Creative Health researchers and practitioners can help functional diversity and promote sustainable wellbeing in the lives of those they support.

Final Thoughts...

This chapter marks the final frame of section two in the Creative Health Communication Framework – 'what is the role of the service-provider.' The four questions explored in this section have demonstrated the various ways that service-providers can clarify their role and enrich the support that they offer to their users. I have explored how the combined stories of participants in this project have unveiled gaps in the language that service-providers use to promote their function. By tracing the consequences of some of these choices, it is possible to consider the importance of including this information within the promotional communication of services. These frames of language help service-providers to differentiate their service from the myriad of competing provisions which are attempting to be seen within the market at present.

Note

1 Re-membering is a Narrative Therapy technique which asks clients to identify the values that were held in their relationship with someone before they died. These values are then used as immortal voices that can live on in the individual's life and allow them to feel the presence of their loved one within their daily experience (Redstone, 2022).

References

Angeler, D.G. and Allen, C.R. (2016) Quantifying resilience. *Journal of Applied Ecology*, 53(3), pp. 617–624.

Bodhi (2022) Interview with Jane Hearst.

De Montfort University (2020) *Research Highlights How Postcodes Impact Children's Career Aspirations*. Available at: https://www.dmu.ac.uk/about-dmu/news/2020/december/research-highlights-how-postcodes-impact-children's-career-aspirations.aspx [Accessed 01/02/2021].

Devan (2021) Interview with Jane Hearst.

Ekundayo (2021) Interview with Jane Hearst.

Gayle (2021) Interview with Jane Hearst.

Gilbert, P. (2009) Introducing compassion-focused therapy. *Advances in Psychiatric Treatment*, 15(3), pp. 199–208.

Hearst, J. (2021) *Aspire to: Children's Book of Representative Role Models*. Leicester: Jane Hearst.

Jiva (2022) Interview with Jane Hearst.

Kris (2021) Interview with Jane Hearst.

Ngoen (2022) Interview with Jane Hearst.

Redstone, A. (2022) *Level 1 Training in Narrative Therapy*. [In-Person Training] The Institute of Narrative Therapy. 3–7 October. Available at: https://www.theint.co.uk/training/level-one/

Winnie (2022) Interview with Jane Hearst.

Stage 3

Contextualising the Service

Chapter 17

The Distinct Roles of Service-User and Service-Provider

In the final section of the Creative Health Communication Framework, I present four frames which look into the context of the service offering. The first of these questions asks whether there is clear communication about the difference between the role of the service-provider and the role of the service-user. This question was developed in response to observations I made during my interviews with participants, whereby they responded differently to the activities depending on their assumptions about my role or expertise as a researcher.

Specifically, some participants followed the activities as they were designed – to elicit personalised conceptualizations of value and build on this through reflective coding. This indicated that these participants were comfortable with a non-structuralist approach to mental wellbeing, whereby a researcher's role is to facilitate exploration of stories and values, rather than apply judgements or frameworks about what they mean (Hayward, 2022). Interestingly, these participants were more likely to either come to the interview expecting it to carry some of the benefits on an intervention or leave feeling like they had gained these benefits consequently. Other participants preferred to tell non-specific stories, with the assumption that I was most qualified to unravel their implicit meanings and code their relevance to mental wellbeing discourse. These participants were more likely to refer to concepts of what a scientific study is designed to achieve, whereby a strict reading of data would be applied via a structuralist lens. Within structuralist theory, mental health professionals are considered the specialist, and members of the public are viewed as cases to organise, make sense of, and fix (Hayward, 2022). White (1997) proposed that this distinction between the role of a helping service-provider and their service-user, in different models of psychology, is best understood in terms of 'centred' and 'decentred' practice. In centred (structuralist) practice, the service-provider's knowledge is at the core of the relationship, with all information being interpreted through this lens. Comparatively, decentred (non-structuralist) practice removes the service-provider from the service-users' stories, with the stories – as they are described by the user – being the best version of truthiness available at that moment.

DOI: 10.4324/9781003423317-24

Hayward (2022) explains that structuralism has been used within dominant western discourse about mental health and wellbeing since Freud introduced layered metaphors to the field in 1909. Naturally, this discourse penetrated the communication and conceptualisation of wellbeing perceived by many members of the public. For service-users who come to a service with these conceptualizations in mind, it will be useful for service-providers to communicate whether this aligns with their own philosophy of wellbeing or not. For services, such as Narrative Therapy, which primarily utilise a decentred approach within their practice, it is possible that their service-users will either need to be guided towards non-structural ways of thinking, or that the service-providers must be willing to adapt around users' requests for more structural elements to be included. For structuralist practitioners, such as Diagnostic Psychiatrists, it may be beneficial to ask clients whether a centred approach is meaningful for them, ahead of the delivery of care. Redstone (2022) explains that centred approaches, which are not endorsed by this user, are at risk of being 'non-influential,' as users' values have not been sown into the diagnostic assessment so do not provide necessary motivation for change.

By exploring some of the examples that were presented during interviews, this section of the framework seeks to demonstrate the impact that users' preconceptions can have on the delivery of care and why, therefore, communication about this may be beneficial for the user-provider relationship.

How Participants' Expectations Shape the Outputs of Research or a Service

Within Lou's interviews, the participant shared a vast array of stories from their life. However, they did not tailor these stories strongly around the activities I have designed. Lou (2021) started with stories that linked to the activities and then shared additional stories that they were reminded of, rather than offering explicit details and observations about the initial story. Lou labelled themselves as a storyteller and explained that the stories they were sharing with me were ones that they have enjoyed telling their friends and acquaintances. Since my recruitment strategy for the project involved going to community groups and asking them if they were interested in sharing their stories with me, Lou had come to the interview with a specific idea of how these stories would be shared based on their past experiences. When telling stories to their friends, who carry similar lifeworld's to their own, Lou could assume that the meaning within their stories was implicit. I attempted to draw the stories closer to the context of the activities, whereby Lou would have a more active hand in coding their own stories, but Lou continued to prefer a free-flowing storytelling style and maintained their assumption that I could unearth the important meaning within these stories based on my perceived role as an expert researcher. Should a research participant or service-user engage like this with a wellbeing service, it would be particularly important to clarify the purpose of the user-provider relationship. If the providers role was to assist Lou in finding unexplored meaning within their stories, then Lou's cyclic storytelling style may need to be managed. Whereas, if the service-provider was led by Lou's desires from the service, it may be that the wellbeing benefits that Lou perceives within storytelling involve the joy of the telling itself.

My observations from this interview, among others who were more structurally inclined, demonstrated a strong alignment to normative social discourses in the UK. This alignment to normative discourses might indicate why they perceive their stories to be easily interpreted and why they are comfortable to have their stories interpreted by a western structuralist framework. Normative social discourse has a strong link to structuralist approaches to care, as both presume there is a right way to live and that individuals should strive for this. With this in mind, another reason structuralism/non-structuralism this is important for Creative Health providers to consider, is within interactions with marginalised demographics. This may include people with recognised protected characteristics or respond to the natural deviations that occur from globalisation and technology-influenced social groupings.

Revisiting Characters Models and Guiding Principles

In Chapter 15, I introduced the distinction between people who rely on character models to inform their actions and those who rely of guiding principles. This showed that some people identify themselves based on identity labels – such as those used to describe different demographics or normative social roles – whereas others carry a more flexible approach centred around value negotiation.

My observations suggest that participants like Lou – who favoured more normative telling of stories – were more likely to describe their stories in relation to their perceived character or social role. For service-providers who wish to reach service-users like these, they may benefit from using a traditional demographic approach to promotion. This approach assumes assimilation of service-users based on one of their identity labels. Services can either engage with shared values associated with these labels or invite service-users to challenge them. For example, a wellbeing service which supports new parents might encourage participants to celebrate their decision to attend a class about how they can become a good parent, or the provider might challenge their user's perceptions of what a 'good' parent looks like by exploring the unique needs of both the child and their parent.

Other participants associated more strongly with the idea of having a guiding principle. These are distinct from identity conceptualisations that are goal orientated as they do not have a desired end or a single point of perfection that can be reached. Instead, they are an adaptive tool which invites the individual to continually reflect on the relationship between their values and their social contexts, evolving with the individual rather than existing counter to their evolving needs. Kris is a good example of someone that applies guiding principles. They demonstrated a clear long-term vision for optimising their life, which referred to self-love and growth as the guiding principles. Moreover, they actively engaged with identifying role-models with similar values to them so that they could refer to their decisions as further guidance on how to apply the principle (Kris, 2021). Throughout their stories, Kris demonstrated a significant deviation from normative ways of living, which they developed as a protective response to traumas. The benefit of adopting this non-structuralist (guiding principles) approach to wellbeing is that it situates wellbeing as a long-term investment rather than a short-term goal. For service-providers who seek to engage with longer-term provisions of care, guiding principles might find a place within their promotional material. Moreover, this approach to promotion is particularly inclusive of intersectional identities as it does not compare their values to dominant discourse, instead opting to celebrate their unique choices and identity. Examples of where this has been applied within existing promotions has been where service-users are invited to 'bring their whole self' rather than the role associated to one of their demographics (Robbins, 2018; Fletcher, 2021; Forbes Council, 2022).

For other users, they may have combined notions of who they are and what they value. For example, Winnie viewed themselves both as a member of their religion – a character with a specific role attached to it – and as an advocate for ethical lifestyles – a guiding principle (Winnie, 2022). Likewise, Jiva's conceptualisation of self lay somewhere in-between a character model and a guiding principle. For example, Jiva said that they aim to engage in selfless and inspiring activities – two guiding principles – but their definition of selflessness and inspiring were both informed by their religion and held particular implications for their role in their local and/or ethnic communities (Jiva, 2022). These scenarios demonstrate that promotional material does not have to be an either-or, but that this content communicates decisions that have an impact on the type of service-users which may be drawn towards a provision.

The Communication of Power

Other concerns, relating to structuralism/non-structuralism and the distinction of roles within the user-provider relationship, is related to the communication of power. For example, within the interviews, my research applied a non-structuralist approach to data collection, as the intention was to develop new insights. Despite this power dynamic being made explicit through the invitation for participants to change activity labels, co-design the meaning of these labels, and to code their own data, notions of structuralism were apparent in participants responses. For example, when Ngoen filed their wellbeing factors into different wellbeing orientations, I asked Ngoen to explain their coding decisions. Ngoen initially interpreted this as my way of communicating disagreement. I, on the other hand, intended only to better understand Ngoen's point of view and prompt more detailed reflection. Similar power relations are likely to exist within the delivery of services, so communication at the commencement of a service is vitally important. The promotion of service values extends beyond marketing material into the service delivery space. Within the context of a service delivery, service-provider's communication style will affect how values are perceived by users, so service-providers benefit from considering how power relations can be communicated about more explicitly ahead of user engagement, and how they are reinforced within sessions to avoid defaulting to other philosophical standpoints.

This mastering of language can be particularly difficult to achieve during scenarios where service-providers must prompt their users. For example, both Winnie and Jiva relied on me to support the research activities with additional prompts. Winnie benefited from the prompts to gauge the scope of inquiry and to generate ideas (Winnie, 2022). Jiva, on the other hand, expressed a simplicity of narrative within the activity responses, but was able to add details during a post-activity conversation (Jiva, 2022). Consequently, service-providers may benefit from including questions within their promotional communication; both ahead of service delivery and within it.

Power relations are inherently at play within the user-provider relationship. In the absence of communication about the difference between the role of the service-provider and that of the service-user, users may fall back on normative ways of conceiving wellbeing interactions. Intentional communication, therefore, either aids the dismantling of these pre-conceptions or strengthens the reasons to engage with them. Moreover, it manages the expectations of service-users and allows them to either search for the most suitable service for their needs or aid them in a negotiation of these values. This will ultimately shape user satisfaction which, in turn, may impact the success the service can achieve via peer-to-peer promotion.

To demonstrate how power-relations can be negotiated and made explicit, I provide a hypothetical example. In this example I demonstrate how service-providers can be explicit in how they perceive mental wellbeing conditions/experiences and invite the user in to negotiate this conceptualisation. I also show how a provider can indicate their role and the role of others in a support group, by attaching these roles to the conceptualisation of mental wellbeing.

> **Service-provider:** Hi Amanda, welcome to our crafts group for people with ADHD! In these sessions, I like to work from a neurodivergence model of ADHD, rather than a deficit model. This means that our sessions will be using craft-making exercises to explore and celebrate our differences, and I'll be referring to society as being disabling rather than humans as disabled. I just wanted to check with you, first, whether you

were comfortable with me talking about your ADHD in this way, as I appreciate that for some people the deficit model resonates and allows their struggles to feel seen.

Service-user (Amanda): Oh, I love the sound of that! I'm happy for you to talk about my ADHD that way, but is it ok for me to still refer to some of the struggles I am experiencing?

Service-provider: Absolutely! These struggles are a very real part of our experience. The neurodivergence model helps us to see that the way our brains work is not wrong, it's just different to how the norms of society expect us to be. But since there are differences there, we will experience a lot of struggles and it's important for you to talk about any that you feel comfortable sharing with the group. You're unlikely to be the only one of us that have experienced some of your struggles, so the peer side of our crafts workshop can be a great way to validate them and hear tips from others that have experienced the same!

The Role of the Service-User/Provider in Creative Health

The reason why I have felt it necessary to touch upon the differences between structuralist and non-structuralist ways of working is because it demonstrates a key distinction between traditional methods of supporting mental health and Creative Health approaches to mental health and wellbeing. Artistic practitioners often favour non-structuralist ways of working. This necessitates the creation of new norms and procedures, along with quality communication about what these procedures look like to those who interact with the service.

One great example of this is an organisation called *Designs in Mind* who are based in Oswestry, Shropshire. Designs in Mind choose to refer to their service-users as artists/members. They believe that the presence of artistic activity naturally leads to improved wellbeing, reduced isolation, and better peer-to-peer support. Consequently, there is no need to position the service-providers as being distinct specialists who hold more power in the relationship. Instead, members are treated as part of a collaborative team, whereby they decide together what to create. The artistic outputs that result from Designs in Mind are turned into sellable pieces of home décor. These pieces are sold both in their local shop and via high profile partnerships. One of the key takeaways that Designs in Mind have observed through this method of interaction, is that participants gain a real sense of fulfilment, as the service repositions the art making away from a label of therapeutic action towards purposeful creation. They believe that in the absence of this power dynamic, whereby members are celebrated for all the skills and creativity that they bring, the wellbeing benefits they receive would not be as great. Another value that Designs in Mind hold is that participating artists are able to have ongoing membership if they please. This encourages a sense of community, rather than treating members as individuals who are only important to interact with when they are unwell. This is one of the methods of interaction in which wellbeing measures move away from symptom and deficit towards a measure of assets. Members often go on to become facilitators, as new members join the community, creating a sense of togetherness, growth and equality. This service, whilst non-structuralist in its format, is linked to other organisational cultures via healthcare structures such as social prescribing. The reason why this frame is so important for context like these is because service-users will find themselves moving from a structuralist system into a non-structuralist community. The ability for a service-provider to communicate their values effectively becomes necessary in these circumstances in order to distinguish themselves from traditional practices and, therefore, attain the outcomes that are uniquely related to their method of working.

Another great example of a decentred working style is Integrated Neighbourhood Working. According to Nottingham and Nottinghamshire Integrated Care System (ICS):

> Successful Integrated Neighbourhood Working (INW) happens when local councils, health and social care, community groups and voluntary sector organisations work together with communities to find ways to improve the health and wellbeing of local people.
>
> (Nottingham and Nottinghamshire ICS, 2024)

For some people this is considered a Creative Health approach as this way of working is a new and innovative way of conceptualising healthcare – particularly as it pertains to power dynamics. One initiative that delivers work following an INW model is Leicester's Community Connectors.

> Community Connectors, was an initiative delivered by Mental Health Matters in 2024. It aimed to reduce isolation and loneliness, improve people's physical and mental wellbeing, and reduce health inequalities. The team was embedded into neighbourhoods, helping to identify provisions, work with members of the community to identify gaps in what was available, and enable the development of new community groups. CreativeHealth activities were included in these developments.
>
> (Hearst, 2025, p.16)

What is particularly interesting about this initiative is that members of the public are empowered to identify their own wellbeing needs *and* the community activities that they would most prefer. This switches around the relationship that service-users have with the provisions available to them. Instead of looking for what exists in the market, and then attending the best match out of that selection, individuals have the power to respond to gaps in the market and request an even more compatible community group. This might be based on preferred hobbies, the type of demographic that they expect to see at this type of activity, or the compatibility of this community group with their culture and ways of thinking. This way of delivering services may be the key to tackling health inequalities across the UK – an area that is particularly of interest to health systems at present due to the strength of research linking social deprivation to decreases in health.

Final Thoughts...

This chapter has chosen to focus on the difference between structuralist and non-structuralist ways of working. The essence of what I am discussing is the importance of communicating what a relationship is intended to look like between researcher and researched or service-user and service-provider. Traditional services often have procedures in place which are there to safeguard both the service-user and service-provider. For example, a therapist may communicate to their clients that their role of supporting the individual is limited to the paid time spent together in the counselling room. Where the arts offer a more fluid approach to mental health and wellbeing care, this act of safeguarding becomes increasingly important. Knowing where the boundaries are between responsibilities is imperative in this fluid space as, in the absence of this communication, service-users are at greater risk of misunderstanding what they can expect from the relationship. Moreover, Creative Health practitioners could be at risk of overstretching their working capacity. This is not good for either their wellbeing all the wellbeing of those they support. As we begin to think about how we can support Creative Health practitioners, to the same degree that medical practitioners are already supported, this consideration of boundaries and power relations is instrumental. In the chapters that follow, I will continue to consider the relationship between service-user and service-provider.

References

Fletcher, P. (2021) *Hard-Headed Truths about 'Bringing Your Whole Self to Work'.* [Online] Entrepreneur. Available at: https://www.entrepreneur.com/leadership/hard-headed-truths-about-bringing-your-whole-self-to-work/384484 [Accessed 01/10/2021].

Forbes Council (2022) *Council Post: 13 Effective Ways To Bring Your 'Whole Self' To Work.* [Online] Forbes. Available at: https://www.forbes.com/sites/forbescoachescouncil/2022/08/10/14-effective-ways-to-bring-your-whole-self-to-work/ [Accessed 21/11/2022].

Hayward, M. (2022) *Level 1 Training in Narrative Therapy.* [In-Person Training] The Institute of Narrative Therapy. 3–7 October. Available at: https://www.theint.co.uk/training/level-one/

Hearst, J. (2025) *Creative Health in the Leicester, Leicestershire and Rutland ICS Region*. Nottingham: The National Centre for Creative Health.
Jiva (2022) Interview with Jane Hearst.
Kris (2021) Interview with Jane Hearst.
Lou (2021) Interview with Jane Hearst.
Nottingham and Nottinghamshire ICS (2024) *Integrated Neighbourhood Working Update*. [Online] Integrated Care System Nottingham and Nottinghamshire. Available at: https://healthandcarenotts.co.uk/integrated-neighbourhood-working-update/ [Accessed 23/10/2024].
Redstone, A. (2022) *Level 1 Training in Narrative Therapy*. [In-Person Training] The Institute of Narrative Therapy. 3–7 October. Available at: https://www.theint.co.uk/training/level-one/
Robbins, M. (2018) *Bring Your Whole Self to Work: How Vulnerability Unlocks Creativity, Connection, and Performance*. Carlsbad, California: Hay House, Inc.
White, M. (1997) *Narratives of Therapists' Lives*. Adelaide, S.A.: Dulwich Centre Publications.
Winnie (2022) Interview with Jane Hearst.

Chapter 18

Single Service or Collaborative Team

In the second frame of section three, I ask the question: *will the service-provider be contributing to a set of collaborative support services or will they be supporting the service-user alone?* This question responds to participant stories which identified multiple, co-occurring threats to wellbeing or described a multifaceted response to previous traumas. Their stories showed that wellbeing experiences are dynamic expressions. In these expressions, some areas of our being can be thriving whilst other areas are struggling. By recognising this dynamic nature, I extrapolate that for people experiencing multiple struggles at the same time, it may be necessary to respond with multiple support services. The interview activities highlighted just how debilitating cumulative negative burdens can be when met with inadequate or misaligned support.

Using the Creative Health Communication Framework to Identify the Need for Collaboration

For service-providers considering whether their place is within a collaborative team or as a sole provider, the answers to the frames explored so far offer a helpful guide. For example, where the service-user has already identified the issue that they seek help with (Chapter 13, frame 5), service-providers offering management services will not need a collaborator to assist with identifying an issue. Likewise, if the service-user's issue clearly resides in either the internal or external world (Chapter 9, frame 1), the service-provider may not need a collaborator to assist with the different aspects of this issue. Similarly, if the issue that the service-user requires is situated within one category of wellbeing (Chapter 11, frame 3), and there is one specific resilience strategy that is most compatible with this issue (Chapter 16, frame 8), then the preciseness of a provider's role begins to become evident. If, on the other hand, a service-user needs some assistance in breaking down their experience and understanding what they require before they make change, they may benefit from having two different support systems in place. If their situation is complex, requiring solutions to multiple interrelated issues that bridge over the

DOI: 10.4324/9781003423317-25

internal and external worlds and require various resilience strategies to solve, then service-providers may want to consider how they manage the scope of their role. One option is to clearly communicate where the boundaries of their support lie and work on managing the ongoing expectations of both them and their user. Alternatively, they may intend to help the bigger picture, but recognise that they will require other specialist skills and assistance for this to be possible.

Replicating and Renovating the Collaborative Approaches of the NHS

For service-providers who wish to work in a team, it may be useful to replicate aspects of the NHS's Care Programme Approach (CPA) which is used by dedicated Mental Health Teams. These teams include different types of specialists, such as psychiatrists, psychologists, community psychiatric nurses, social workers, and occupational therapists. Each member of the team carries a clear role within the collaboration. Sometimes teams are prepared to take on some responsibilities outside of their role during emergency scenarios or in contexts where their involvement is more practical and efficient. These roles are made explicit at the beginning of a team arrangement so that each provider knows when it is their responsibility to assist the service-user or not. The team then work together, using a care plan as a guide to their responsibility and goals.

As social prescribing and non-clinical approaches to health become increasingly accepted into the mental health system, there will be more scope for Creative Health practitioners to be brought into MHTs. If the goal of a Creative Health service-provider is to work alongside other professionals to assist with acute mental health cases, then the use of the Creative Health Communication Framework will be a powerful means of communicating how each stakeholder's role differs from the other members of the team and where the value of their service has a part to play in the patients' recovery.

Alternatively, artistic providers might wish to be part of teams that are not medically focused. For providers who prefer a route which does not pathologize human experiences of poor wellbeing, but still require a team of practitioners to support their goals, it may still prove beneficial to learn from the CPA approach to care. The better service-providers can communicate their shared goals within a team and develop a plan that is attractive to their service-user, the greater the chances are that they will achieve harmony and shared success.

For other service-providers, they may find that they do not need the help of different types of specialists, but the provision they are developing is a collaborative type of art – for example, Filmmaking Therapies. In this case, being able to develop ground rules, along with a communal sense of direction and purpose, is still important. This ensures that everyone within the team recognises that the purpose of the intervention is the wellbeing aspect and that the art itself, no matter how well made, falls secondary to that in importance.

Lessons from Participant Stories

To illustrate the comparison between practitioner-focused care and team-delivered care, stories from participant interviews offer some suggestions of how appropriate care plans might be developed:

Several participants in the interviews expressed comfortingly matter-of-fact explanations of the self. Jiva, for example, said that they are human and that this is all that they were intended to be, adding that they whilst they may aim to leave a legacy of being kind and selfless, these are choices rather than things they should internalise to their detriment (Jiva, 2022). Likewise, Bodhi expressed a fondness for keeping things simple, stating 'I never ever think "am I a good person?," "am I this person?," you know, I just get on with life without actually putting a label on it' (Bodhi, 2022). Equally, Winnie declared, 'It's enough to be remembered. That's how people live on; by being remembered. Hopefully with affection' (Winnie, 2022).

However, this type of control is only possible within a facilitative environment. In experiences like that of Ekundayo, where the chaotic nature of their abuse left their internal world at attention (Ekundayo, 2021), it was not so easy to keep the internal voice simple and unaffected by external threats. Ekundayo spoke of moments where their parent threatened to kill themself, telling every sibling except Ekundayo that they loved them, before locking themself into a room with a knife. They described ongoing tensions, like the fear of getting a drink in case they got shouted at, or the ability of their parent to isolate them from the rest of their family anytime that they were annoyed (Ekundayo, 2021). These psychological mind games may be caused externally, but their internal effects were held far past the moments that they occurred. Once Ekundayo escaped this abusive household, the lasting internal deterioration had a negative causal effect on Ekundayo's decision-making and emotional stability (Ekundayo, 2021).

If a service-provider had a role to uplift an individual's self-esteem through creative exercises, the way that they would approach supporting Ekundayo would vary greatly from their approach to supporting Jiva, Bodhi, and Winnie. For Jiva, Bodhi, and Winnie, these exercises could build upon their foundations of what it means to be human, celebrate the fallibility of humans which is written into these foundations, and ask the participants how they wished to leave a mark on the present day. If the same service-provider sought to support Ekundayo, they might need to consider whether Ekundayo has access to a safe environment and whether the toxic messages indoctrinated by their parent have left behind physiological, perceptual, or behavioural impacts. The provider might offer a service which focused on rewriting their abuse story to one where they became the protagonist and their values mattered the most. They might connect Ekundayo to other peers who have experienced the same, to normalise Ekundayo's experience and provide role models of what is possible. Only once these aspects of Ekundayo's experience had been addressed, could they be deemed to take the same benefits as Jiva, Bodhi, and Winnie from a service.

In this instance, the provider must ask themselves whether these, more complex threats, are still their responsibility to support, or whether they are better served by other specialists. The service-provider can then choose whether they hold any responsibility for developing this collaborative team, or if they can encourage the service-user to engage with more services themselves. Collaborations do not need to be formal partnerships to be successful. Rather, it is important to recognise each service's strength and know when the service-provider is best suited to signpost additional support mechanisms. By using the language afforded throughout the Creative Health Communication Framework, service-providers can support service-users in their mental health literacy and empower them to create a support plan which works for them. Where formal collaborations do exist, then this language can be used to identify gaps in care and can help develop a more effective plan. Moreover, the language is not tailored to one discipline over another, which facilitates an equitable discussion between providers who were typically afforded disproportionate levels of power.

Applying the Learning to Creative Health

During my work at the National Centre for Creative Health, I was responsible for delivering a number of huddle events. Huddles are co-production spaces between people experiencing difficulties with their mental health and wellbeing, the healthcare professionals who seek to support this type of mental health and wellbeing, along with creative practitioners. Using arts or creativity as a facilitation tool, these spaces aim to unearth new insights into a particular health and wellbeing concern or the experiences of a particular demographic. One of the huddle events that I hosted was a collaboration with Headway, the brain injury organisation. At this event I worked with Headway's service-users to explore the Creative Health Communication Framework. The participants shared their stories of living with brain injury and helped to identify the type of support services they benefit from. Headway was interested in exploring where in the service needs there was opportunity to bring more Creative Health into their offering.

One of the observations I was able to make as a consequence of these storytelling events was that Headway offered a comprehensive response to brain injury; one which required an awareness of multiple partners of whom they could signpost their service-users towards. These partners included those responsible for supporting benefits claims. The staff members at Headway held a basic awareness of how they users may rely on benefits and some of the basic legalities which determine which kind of support they were entitled to. The partnering organisations were then able to get into the details of the benefit system, supporting individuals with the unique needs and contexts. The benefits of Headway holding some responsibility for signposting and holding awareness of these external support offers meant that people who accessed Headway's services were able to access additional support they did not know existed previously. This was particularly of use to those who had recently acquired a brain injury, or those who had only recently found out about Headway's offering. In the absence of this collaborative support, individuals were at risk of experiencing family breakdown after the injury, as well as financial strain, increased experiences of depression, and more incidences of loneliness. Headway helps them to reimagine their life as somebody with a brain injury, helping them to enact it not only in theory but via appropriate signposted support. That role in this collaboration is to be the first point of contact for those trying to understand the systems that support this highly specific experience. They also play a key role in providing peer-to-peer support and a place of safety and understanding.

In this collaborative arrangement, Headway does not hold formal ties to all the organisations that it signposts to, in terms of commissioning or mental health care plans. Yet they recognise, from the onset, that the power of their work is only possible within a collaborative landscape. They understand their role and are able to communicate this very clearly with their service-users.

Turning to another example of where collaboration plays a key role in the development of the Creative Health landscape, I briefly discuss some of the systematic provisions that are in place to encourage more integration of healthcare responses. Firstly, across the UK we can see a number of cultural compacts taking an interest in Creative Health (Hearst, 2024). Cultural Compacts play a key role in facilitating cross industry collaboration. This usually involves members of the local councils – often from the cultural teams – as well as leadership from key arts institutions in the area. In some areas, like that of Shropshire Telford and Wrekin, the board of the cultural compact also includes representation from the Integrated Care Board and from Public Health – two key healthcare stakeholders. This demonstrates a commitment to integrating health into the cultural agenda in the region. As we try to bridge the two disparate industries of culture and health, collaborative spaces like that created by the Cultural Compact will become instrumental to the development of a Creative Health scene.

Elsewhere in our systems, we see a movement towards integration of clinical health providers and third sector health and care support. The arts, when used for health and social care purposes, would have traditionally fit in the third sector. However, as we increasingly develop our evidence towards the benefits of the arts towards clinical outcomes, as well as demonstrating the link between preventative health behaviours and long-term health outcomes, there is a rising consensus that the arts should bridge both types of healthcare.

It is important then, that systems are following this path of change towards greater patient voice, more non-clinical services which focus on wicked issues, and greater equality of voice around the healthcare table. Two places where this systematic change is evident, is in the health transformation programmes that are taking place across the UK, along with the legislation which necessitates the presence of an Integrated Care System. These Integrated Care Systems must include a VCSE alliance, whereby voluntary community and social enterprise partners have a say on our developing healthcare.

Final Thoughts...

Whatever the unique mix of wellbeing needs that service-providers are presented with, they can apply the different aspects of the Creative Health Communication Framework to identify a service's value. By knowing the value of their service, providers can be bolder in their delivery and promotion of care and reduce the risk of feeling responsible for a person's entire wellbeing. In a wellbeing climate which experiences a significant amount of burnout by wellbeing professionals (Simpson et al., 2019; Finan, McMahon and Russell, 2022; Davies et al., 2022), these boundaries of care are becoming increasingly important. Recognising the limits of one's ability to support others is an important step in developing robust Creative Health services which can stand up to the rigour of healthcare procurement procedures, safeguard their service-users, and build trust with users. The next chapter will build upon this theme of trust in more detail.

References

Bodhi (2022) Interview with Jane Hearst.

Davies, S.M. et al. (2022) Factors influencing 'burn-out' in newly qualified counsellors and psychotherapists: A cross-cultural, critical review of the literature. *Counselling and Psychotherapy Research*, 22(1), pp. 64–73.

Ekundayo (2021) Interview with Jane Hearst.

Finan, S., McMahon, A. and Russell, S. (2022) "At What Cost am I Doing This?" An interpretative phenomenological analysis of the experience of burnout among private practitioner psychotherapists. *Counselling and Psychotherapy Research*, 22(1), pp. 43–54.

Hearst, J. (2024) *The Impact of Cultural Compacts in Promoting Creative Health Activity*. [Online] The National Centre for Creative Health. Available at: https://ncch.org.uk/blog/the-impact-of-cultural-compacts-in-promoting-creative-health-activity [Accessed 25/06/2024].

Jiva (2022) Interview with Jane Hearst.

Simpson, S. et al. (2019) Burnout amongst clinical and counselling psychologist: The role of early maladaptive schemas and coping modes as vulnerability factors. *Clinical Psychology & Psychotherapy*, 26(1), pp. 35–46.

Winnie (2022) Interview with Jane Hearst.

Chapter 19

Trust-Building and Attainability of Healthcare Services

The question explored in this chapter is, perhaps, the most vital question in section three of the Creative Health Communication Framework. That is, *how does the researcher/service-provider plan to develop trust and make their service more attainable?*

Throughout my interviews, participants shared stories about the attainability of quality support and the mistrust that arises when a service-user is allocated – what they perceived to be – sub-standard support. Here, the word attainability is specifically used to describe barriers – often related to service finances or availability of specialists – which hinder the number of people that can access the support, and the speed at which this support becomes available to them.

Why Trust and Attainability Are Important Considerations

My research demonstrates that mental health services are often oversubscribed (Buchan et al., 2019; NHS England and NHS Improvement, 2020; Palmer et al., 2021) and have long waiting lists (Baker, Canvin and Berzins, 2019). For those that receive care, half of respondents report that the number of sessions was not enough to support their needs (Mind, 2013). Two-fifths of patients waiting for support are forced to resort to emergency or crisis services (Royal College of Psychiatrists, 2020) and there was a 65% rise in demand for private counselling services between 2016 and 2018 (Whyman, 2018). The current cost of living crisis has placed limitations on poorer individuals regarding the attainability of private care, causing them to cancel therapy sessions (BACP, 2022). This, in turn, has meant that access to mental health support has become more readily attained by wealthier users. Participant data added to this picture by demonstrating how services vary in quality, such as the availability and characteristics of counselling support. Moreover, my conversations with artistic service-providers, via networking and events, has built my understanding of arts-specific limitations. One that is often repeated is the time-limited nature of financial support,

DOI: 10.4324/9781003423317-26

whereby project-by-project provisions do not have the time to develop their user-base or meet their full potential.

With this vast array of limitations shaping the wellbeing market offer, it is inevitable that service-users will begin to feel hopeless, disenfranchised, and mistrusting of provisions. This question, therefore, invites researchers and service-providers to engage with research participants and service-users in dialogue about the limitations that services carry, as this accountability recognises the validity of service-users' wellbeing concerns despite the providers' ability to support them. Whilst this transparency will not solve their issue of attaining services, it instigates a journey of redeveloping trust with mental healthcare. Once trust has been redeemed, users may become more comfortable in trying newly formed solutions, such as those proposed by Creative Health specialists. It is particularly important for Creative Health services to attain trust from their users, as these provisions are not as heavily promoted within dominant mental health discourse, so come with a sense of uncertainty. Creative Health service-providers will need to be aware of this sense of uncertainty when promoting their provisions, as they are afforded an opportunity to bring clarity to their promotions and help service-users feel safer, more aware of what their provision can achieve, and how it differs from their experiences elsewhere. To redevelop trust with research participants and service-users, researchers and service-providers should consider the scope of events that inform mistrust and the types of mistrust these events produce.

Systems, Cultures, and Social Influences

Based on the stories I collected from participants, experiences of trust begin in a service-user's lived environment. For instance, where an individual's immediate social network is unsupportive, this can evoke feelings of helplessness during their consideration of whether to search for support through the market. Ngoen, for example, shared how the lack of support they experienced from their ex-partner affected their ability to feel well (Ngoen, 2022). They explained that whilst they did experience support from one of their parents, this alone, was not enough. Here, Ngoen expressed a loneliness in opinion, whereby the lack of support they experienced from their loved ones and peers led them to consider whether support was achievable in their current environment. How service-providers respond to these types of barriers depends entirely on the type of provision they intend to deliver. For a service that promotes liberation or the development of communities of choice, they might choose to build upon their user's outsider status in their promotional narrative. Whereas providers who seek to redevelop the cohesiveness of communities, might opt to celebrate, within their promotional narrative, the values that unite them.

Culture is an important social influence to consider in this exploration of environments and trust. For example, in Samawah's interview (Samawah, 2022) they explained that their wellbeing is affected by cultural taboos and the barriers they create for communication: '[Members of my culture] do not consider mental illnesses or mental events as something important. Physical, yes. Mental, no' (Samawah, 2022). More work is needed to appropriately engage with these barriers and develop conceptualisations of wellbeing that resonate with cultural values, whilst still promoting the value of support.

One of my efforts regarding the Creative Health Communication Framework has been conceptualise mental health literacy as a 'mosaic of different literacies which may be deployed in different settings and in line with different experiences' (Raghavan et al., 2022) rather than prioritise the 'literacy' of the medical industry. By taking the experiences of participants as a guide, the framework acts as a bridge between the mental health literacies of individuals and the literacies of different mental health industries. This bridging language can be used to make users' experiences feel seen and respected – offering them further insights about their wellbeing, on their own terms rather than the terms of medical practitioners. Researchers and service-providers who are interested in using the framework in this way can begin to engage with the agenda of making care inclusive, by consulting members of their target demographics and trialling promotional exercises. Tools exist which can guide these providers through the process of reaching marginalised groups (e.g., Farooqi et al., 2022).

Adding to culture and social environments, systems can also influence an individual's wellbeing. By considering which systems affect wellbeing and how they affect a target demographic, researchers and service-providers can incorporate responses within their promotional narrative. An example of what I mean by systematic influence comes from Aje's interview (Aje, 2022). Aje described an apprehension to using a wellbeing service when they did not perceive themselves to be the most in need of that service. Since the mental health services in the UK prioritise acute mental health needs for the sake of managing waiting lists, it is unsurprising that members of the public internalise this pressure. Important to this, Creative Health services thrive in preventative care. Since the market prioritises responsive care, sometimes to its own detriment, the preventative nature of the arts affords artistic researchers and providers the opportunity for a differentiation-leadership strategy (a strategy discussed in Chapter 2) (Porter, 1980; Porter, 1985). This would entail the field of Creative Health becoming leading advocates of preventative care and promoting their services as exemplars of this. Another appropriate response, at the level of service delivery, entails service-providers managing the expectations of their users. For example, where Aje was able to reflect on their emotions and conclude that they were justified in wanting support, because 'it's easier to be in a space where someone is focused purely on unravelling things' (Aje, 2022), other users may struggle to prioritise their needs in this way. These users benefit from hearing supportive commentary about who is eligible for support and what type of needs can be supported.

To promote the inclusivity of their service, providers can add phrases such as 'no need is too small' to their promotional material.

Quality of Service Delivery

So far, my examples have shown that attainability of support is not always a problem with services alone, but also dependent on our state of mind, programmed associations, and relational dependence. However, there were also examples, within participant stories, which demonstrated the erosion of trust caused by previous service-providers. One of the issues identified within this deterioration of trust is how services within the medical system often rely on the support of primary care providers – namely GP's. When this relationship exhibits issues with discrimination, lack of mental health literacy, or otherwise eroded trust, service-users can feel limited in options if they cannot afford to access private care. An example from participant stories, was through the experience of Devan. They explained:

> My doctor was really not very helpful. You know, everything was in my head. [They] just wanted to give me any old anti-depressants. I kept asking [them] for talking therapies [and their response was] 'no no no no no'. You know. [They] always made me feel like [they] just wanted to get me out the office.
>
> (Devan, 2021)

For providers - like those from the field of Creative Health – who are not subjected to the same NHS limitations, philosophy, or methodological limitations, there is ample opportunity to differentiate themselves from the existing mental wellbeing industry and demonstrate how the arts can be more trust-worthy.

Once Devan had experienced negative interactions like this with their doctor, they carried a mistrust of the doctor and became sceptical of their professionalism more widely. Devan explained that they believe their GP has a drinking problem and that the doctor could be seen walking around the neighbourhood with alcohol in their hand (Devan, 2021). This demonstrates that trust in the user-provider relationship extends beyond the hours of primary care, across any interactions shared between the user and the provider. Accordingly, professionalism and approachability must be carefully negotiated within different types of communication.

If values of confidentiality, being unjudgmental, exemplary, and of trustworthy mind, are all important attributes of a medical professional, then this must also be true for Creative Health professionals. Whilst the behaviour at the centre of Devan's criticism is beyond the scope of this book about language, there are ways of indicating professionalism within the stories and language that are used within promotions.

One place where potential conflicts relating to our understanding of professionalism may rise is in relation to anti-discrimination movements. Many emerging Creative Health providers seek to decolonise, declass, or otherwise remove discrimination from systems of care, using accessible role-models and language. The challenge, here, is in balancing these anti-discriminatory sentiments with stories that can elicit professionalism-related trust. Where researchers and service-providers seek to avoid over-professionalising their role – i.e., they want to emphasise equal power relations between user and provider – they can exemplify their quality of practice by demonstrating their values outside of the helping environment and/or sharing personal experiences which they believe offer participants insight into the type of problem they are supporting. These expressions make clear the value they attribute to users' experiences and wellbeing goals and manage the expectations of where they fit within this journey to inspire trust in their users.

Another thing to respond to within this consideration of trust is the negative experiences that users might associate with artists. This might be responded to by challenging stereotypes or being clearer about the role of a service, or there might be a genuine safe-guarding concern. Devan, for example, shared:

> I've met a lot of narcissistic and sociopathic – even the odd psychopathic – person in my life. […] There's a lot of those kind of people in the arts. And, you know, I've had some very unpleasant experiences with some of them. (Devan, 2021)

As researchers and service-providers develop their work and choose potential collaborators, it is important to consider how they will safeguard their service-users against foul-play, and how this is communicated to service-users so that they can develop trust. This may involve the creation of rules that can be shared between collaborators and service-users and signed to agree their shared respect. This holds each person accountable and puts safeguarded boundaries into the relationship. Service-providers working in large teams may choose to create a grievance procedure, which is clearly communicated via FAQ's or a contract. Or, if they are working alone, they may have a communication framework in place to manage conflict. This ensures that the wellbeing needs of both the service-user and the service-provider is balanced. Having these systems in place is fundamental to offering security for both the provider and their service-user, even if the delivery of their provision itself seeks to be structurally adaptable. Counselling principles can be a useful reference in the development of Creative Health safeguarding procedures. An example is where therapists agree the terms of their relationship within their initial consultation. This agreement covers expectations, such as the time allocation of responsibility.

One of the benefits of outlining the role of a service-provider, in the manner encouraged through this framework, is that the scope of their responsibility is more clearly outlined, based on specific threats they are supporting and a specific method of supporting this threat. These distinctions can benefit service-users who engage in group activities. For example, if a Creative Health researcher or service-provider were to encourage shared storytelling and inter-group care within a defined space, it does not become the responsibility of these participants to follow these expectations outside of the service space. By being clear with these distinctions, the service-provider allows the user to feel supported and this will increase their ability to reach out if another user burdens them with too much responsibility. The type of trust afforded to service-users, in this case, is not trust in the service-provider per say, but trust in the boundaries of the service.

The Wider Healthcare Industry

Elsewhere in participant interviews, stories of mistrust were not always in relation to the mental health industry but were impacted by other health and support systems including Support Workers, Dentists, and Social Service Staff. This demonstrates that there is a breadth of professional influences that can shape a service-users' trust or apathy. Consequently, there are benefits of distinguishing Creative Health services from these experiences.

One example was Ekundayo's experience of being let down by social services as a child. This story told of Ekundayo's parent hitting Ekundayo's sibling and 'bashing' their head on the side of a table (Ekundayo, 2021). After many failed attempts to build up courage, these siblings finally reported their parent to social services. When social services came round, the parent said the story was fictitious and blamed Ekundayo for 'doing theatre' (Ekundayo, 2021). The social services team left having not spoken to the children themselves, who were ready to divulge more information. This account shaped the children's courage and affected their trust in the years that followed. Ekundayo felt like either nobody cared enough about their pain, or these people were defenceless against their parent's manipulations (Ekundayo, 2021). This example demonstrates how trust can be impacted between support services, as this lack of acknowledgement contributed towards Ekundayo 'feeling insane' from living the life they knew to be true and playing the life that other people wanting to be true. They explained that a consequence of this was that they had struggled to recognise the degree to which they could classify this as abuse until after they left the family home and accessed therapy (Ekundayo, 2021).

In cases where Creative Health service-providers wish to serve disenfranchised users, like Ekundayo, they may benefit from using promotional language which positions the provider as an ally. This may involve mirroring users' own words and expressions back to them, to pay recognition to their own understanding and agency (Hayward, 2022). Alternatively, it might involve explicitly calling out inappropriate behaviour, or aligning via educational content online. Another consideration might be the privacy of promotional communication – for example, service-providers may situate themselves within attainable reach of a user whilst keeping their services low-profile for anyone that may cause harm to a vulnerable individual. These considerations begin to exceed the scope of a language framework, but are still relevant to promotional communication in terms of visibility of promotion to the general population.

Disenfranchisement

Developing this topic of trust-building, it is important for service-providers to also consider how the delivery of services can lead to feelings of disenfranchisement, as market concerns, such as financial restraints, shape services. One key example involves the digitalisation of healthcare, which has left pockets of the population with barriers to access (Morris and Brading, 2007; Lupton, 2014; Ibrahim et al., 2021). Whilst this is not an issue with trust, in a traditional manner, it does shape a user's confidence in interacting with a service and their sense of being understood.

This barrier was explicit in Winnie's story (Winnie, 2022), as their doctor now asks for photos of Winnie's problems before in-person appointments are made available. As an individual with barriers associated with digital literacy, this requirement to know how to take a photo prevents Winnie from receiving any care. Winnie concluded that these practices are 'creating barriers to living' and that they complicate an already messy system of care (Winnie, 2022). Creative Health providers who are aware of issues like this, can communicate about them within their service promotion. If they offer a service that does not rely on technology, then they can describe how this makes it more accessible to demographics who have a lack of digital literacy or a barrier to accessing technology. If the service does engage with technology, then the arts provider benefits from including information about what type of digital literacy is required from their users. Depending on their strengths, the provider could also communicate the benefits that they can offer, such as easier access to appointments, a faster delivery of care, or an ethos of putting the client first.

Responding to Stigma and Worries about Burden

A final area that influenced participants willingness to engage with support services was their perceptions on stigma and burden. Many participants, for example, included dialogue or subject matter within their interview that they worried may be ill-received – whether it be deemed a social faux pas or politically incorrect. All these participants, upon receiving my positive affirmation, were able to continue their commentary in full and thanked me for my ability to focus on the intention behind words and stories. However, this information may not have been readily shared in other settings, demonstrating the importance of facilitation style. By considering the cultures associated with generations, ethnicities, and communities, along with the social discourses and communication styles this exposes the individual to, researchers and service-providers can enter the collaboration space with openness and grace. This not only harnesses understanding, but also opens opportunities for this language to be comfortably negotiated, if necessary.

Adding to this, other participants commented that they were continuously reflecting on how much was safe to share, with my own wellbeing being a key concern. These concerns were rooted in ideas about how much other people should share responsibility for mental wellbeing, with participants viewing their stories as a burden rather than an insight. All shared more than they expected to when they were coming into the session – even those who decided there was a particular topic they did not want to discuss in detail. The concerns associated with facilitator burden indicate two engagement barriers for people receiving mental health and wellbeing support: 1) worries that they will be forced to talk about something they do not wish to share or 2) fears about being or becoming a burden. Service-providers who are offering relevant provisions may wish to include information in their promotional material detailing the right to omit details that the users are not comfortable with sharing. Likewise, they might include information about the support mechanisms that a provider has in place, which makes them able to take the full brunt of a service-user's problems within the designated session. Elsewhere, providers choose to communicate the boundaries of their responsibility, such as it only being the provider's burden during the hours of the service. This functions, both to protect the provider and comfort the user, by knowing where their responsibilities lie and burden ends. This allows the user to gain trust, reduce anxiety, and make an informed decision about whether this service is suited to them.

Attainability and Trust in Creative Health

A great example of how creative services have sought to make their offering more attainable comes from The Wellcome Collection, a free museum and library in London/online that explores the past, present and future of health. As part of their offering, Wellcome offers relaxed openings of their exhibitions to make them more user-friendly for neurodivergent audiences. In their advertisements for these relaxed openings, Wellcome is explicit about the target audience of neurodivergent people. They then briefly outline what type of stories appear throughout the exhibition, to aid with expectation management and emotional modelling. They then share a photo of what the space looks like at the beginning of the exhibition, with some information of how to get to this space. Again, this helps with predictive modelling and allows neurodivergent people to reduce feelings of anxiety. Next, Wellcome explain some of the features in the exhibit that have particular sensory qualities that could be attractive or overstimulating to different people who are neurodivergent. For example, in the exhibit *Jason and the Adventure of 254* (Wellcome Collection, 2024). Wellcome explain that there are sculptures that can be touched, dioramas that light up when you press a button, and many illustrations to look at. They also provide a small selection of photos that indicate how bright the exhibition colours are. Finally, they outline what extra provisions are available on the relaxed opening days. This includes extra staff available to help, fewer visitors and more space, sensory support equipment such as ear defenders, tinted glasses and stim toys, comfortable cushions and mats, and a chill out space. The range of dates available for relaxed openings is plentiful, signalling to neurodivergent audiences that they are genuinely welcome, considered and cared about.

Initiatives like Wellcome's relaxed openings are becoming more commonplace. Examples include the work of Stims Collective, a group of autistic film scholars, journalists, and filmmakers, who create and curate accessible and relaxed spaces for neurodiverse audiences. Their relaxed screenings can entail a number of accessibility-related actions, including unassigned seating with plenty of space, house lights slightly dimmed but not turned off, film volume turned slightly down, freedom to move around and make noise, and a signposted quiet area near the auditorium (Stims Collective, 2024). Another great example of how creativity has been made more attainable for neurodivergent audiences includes *Kaleidoscopic Realms* (Nottingham Castle, 2024), an installation of artworks by eight contemporary artists on the theme of intuitive mark-marking in its many forms. As part of the exhibition, the team created special measures to make it attainable to audiences with addition needs. This included a session with Sarah Marsh, where attendees were invited to wrap themselves in soft, tactile sculptural objects and wear these as they walked around the displays. These relaxed viewings were also quieter, with less attendees, lower lighting levels throughout, where staff were trained to support people with additional support needs. Finally, neurodivergent audiences are not the only demographic that service-providers may choose to focus on in making their work/spaces more attainable. Applying similar principles to make art more accessible to people of colour and/or working-class audiences, Saziso Phiri create the Anti-Gallery. The Anti-Gallery takes art out of traditional gallery environments, to more familiar and comfortable spaces. Saziso explains to Left Lion magazine:

> I think art galleries are very important but they do have issues. I have conversations with people who wouldn't usually go into a gallery space for various reasons – sometimes they feel it's intimidating or that it's only for the elite. What I want to do is help break down those barriers, or at least blur the lines, and get people interested in engaging with art.
>
> (Vaughan, 2017)

Similar to these initiatives, a great example of where providers have implemented actions that develop trust comes from Leicester City Council (LCC). LCC has a team within its public health department which coordinates a programme called Community Champions. These are members of the community and community organisations who are able to influence their local populations as a trusted and integrated leader. The format of the Community Champions initiative means that there is a necessary two-way relationship between the council and the community leaders. Leaders are able to respond to the council with insights and opinions they have gathered from their local neighbourhood and shape the priorities of healthcare in the area. They are also able to offer understanding into the barriers that people from the area perceive or experience. This was crucial for the delivery of complex health responses, such as the vaccination rollout during covid. One of the things that was highlighted at this time was the importance of having community leaders who can communicate to people in their first language. This aids comprehension about the risks and rewards of different health behaviours and interventions, improving the interaction of members of the public with things that support their health and wellbeing.

Final Thoughts...

With these various considerations about trust and attainability in mind, I conclude that providers of Creative Health services benefit from considering the status of an individual as they first encounter promotional material, and when they first engage with a service. In cases where there is an erosion of trust in traditional systems, Creative Health researchers and service-providers may wish to emphasise how they differ in their approaches – whereby user voice is often put more centre stage. However, where users are comforted by the structure and specialism of traditional services, emphasis on the professionalism of Creative Health services may be key to building trust. This is a fine balance that should be appropriately considered ahead of research engagement or service delivery, so that expectations can be managed.

The Creative Health sector comes with its own shortcomings, so trustful communication is not limited to resolving issues of the past but also arming against potential future conflicts of interest. For example, Creative Health services are often underfunded or run on a project-by-project basis; in this case, providers may wish to consider how they communicate the reasons why interested individuals are not able to participate, or signpost them to other provisions. They might wish to decide among their teams how this is communicated to interested parties, so that they retain the confidence to ask another programme for help. This might be via the traditional signposting to emergency support agencies. However, this runs the risk of delegitimising their experience if they do not view it as extreme or aligned to those support services. A way to encourage the exploration of any type of wellbeing journey may involve more conversational time, encouragement to find their own resources, sprinkled with insights the provider may have of the industry in the form of top tips.

By communicating the strengths and limitations of their service, Creative Health providers prevent negative associations from being created by users with misaligned needs, who may have benefitted more from being signposted elsewhere. Here, services are not always in competition with each other, in the way typically encouraged by a market, rather, they are part of a joint mission to improve wellbeing that is shaped by the need to simultaneously survive as a business entity.

References

Aje (2022) Interview with Jane Hearst.

BACP (2022) *Cost of Living Crisis: Survey Shows Impact on Mental Health*. Available at: https://www.bacp.co.uk/news/news-from-bacp/2022/8-september-cost-of-living-crisis-survey-shows-impact-on-mental-health/ [Accessed 04/10/2022].

Baker, J.A., Canvin, K. and Berzins, K. (2019) The relationship between workforce characteristics and perception of quality of care in mental health: A qualitative study. *International Journal of Nursing Studies*, 100, p. 103412.

Buchan, J. et al. (2019) A critical moment: NHS staffing trends, retention and attrition. *The Health Foundation*, p. 38. Available at: https://www.health.org.uk/sites/default/files/upload/publications/2019/A%20Critical%20Moment_1.pdf [Accessed 18/08/2020].

Devan (2021) Interview with Jane Hearst.

Ekundayo (2021) Interview with Jane Hearst.

Farooqi, A. et al. (2022) Developing a toolkit for increasing the participation of black, Asian and minority ethnic communities in health and social care research. *BMC Medical Research Methodology*, 22(1), p. 17.

Hayward, M. (2022) *Level 1 Training in Narrative Therapy*. [In-Person Training] The Institute of Narrative Therapy. 3–7 October. Available at: https://www.theint.co.uk/training/level-one/

Ibrahim, H. et al. (2021) Health data poverty: An assailable barrier to equitable digital health care. *The Lancet Digital Health*, 3(4), pp. e260–e265.

Lupton, D. (2014) Critical perspectives on digital health technologies. *Sociology Compass*, 8(12), pp. 1344–1359.

Mind (2013) *We Still Need to Talk A Report on Access to Talking Therapies*. London: Mind.

Morris, A. and Brading, H. (2007) E-literacy and the grey digital divide: A review with recommendations. *Journal of Information Literacy*, 1(3), pp. 13–28.

Ngoen (2022) Interview with Jane Hearst.

NHS England and NHS Improvement (2020) *Managing Capacity and Demand Within Inpatient and Community Mental Health, Learning Disabilities and Autism Services for All Ages*. London: NHS England. Available at: https://www.england.nhs.uk/coronavirus/wp-content/uploads/sites/52/2020/03/C0841-managing-demand-and-capacity-across-mh-and-ld-v2.pdf

Nottingham Castle (2024) *Kaleidoscopic Realms*. [Online] Nottingham Castle. Available at: https://www.nottinghamcastle.org.uk/kaleidoscopic-realms/ [Accessed 22/10/2024].

Palmer, W. et al. (2021) *Untapped? Understanding the Mental Health Clinical Support Workforce*. London: Nuffield Trust.

Porter, M.E. (1980) *Competitive Strategy: Techniques for Analyzing Industries and Competitors*. New York: Free Press.

Porter, M.E. (1985) *Competitive Advantage: Creating and Sustaining Superior Performance*. New York: London: Free Press; Collier Macmillan.

Raghavan, R. et al. (2022) Multiple mental health literacies in a traditional temple site in Kerala: The intersection between beliefs, spiritual and healing regimes. *Culture, Medicine, and Psychiatry*. [Online] Available at: https://doi.org/10.1007/s11013-022-09800-6 [Accessed 20/11/2022].

Royal College of Psychiatrists (2020) *Two-fifths of Patients Waiting for Mental Health Treatment Forced to Resort to Emergency or Crisis Services*. London: Royal College of Psychiatrists.

Samawah (2022) Interview with Jane Hearst.

Stims Collective (2024) *Relaxed Screenings*. [Online] Stims. Available at: https://www.stims.uk/relaxed-events [Accessed 22/10/2024].

Vaughan, L.J. (2017) *The Anti Gallery*. [Online] Left Lion. Available at: https://leftlion.co.uk/features/2017/02/the-anti-gallery/ [Accessed 22/10/2024].

Wellcome Collection (2024) *Jason and the Adventure of 254*. [Online] Welcome Collection. Available at: https://wellcomecollection.org/exhibitions/jason-and-the-adventure-of-254 [Accessed 22/10/2024].

Whyman, C. (2018) *Increased Demand for Private Counsellors | MHS*. [Online] MHT. Available at: https://www.mentalhealthtoday.co.uk/news/awareness/rise-in-demand-for-private-counsellors-as-patients-say-nhs-waiting-lists-are-too-long [Accessed 21/11/2022].

Winnie (2022) Interview with Jane Hearst.

Chapter 20

Promotional Voices

Scientific, Storytelling, or Poetic

In this chapter, I discuss the question: *can the researcher/service-provider identify the appropriate 'voice' to discuss tangible or intangible resources?* This question responds to the tensions between scientific and artistic providers, whereby superficial hierarchies are created relating to how information is shared. Referring to participant stories, I demonstrate how there are three distinct voices that are available when promoting health-benefitting services, such as Creative Health activities. These voices are scientific, storytelling, and poetic. They are each shaped by the tangibility of the resource being offered.

I believe that different communication styles work better for different contexts. Accordingly, I demonstrate how these three voices can be applied to a single, hypothetical provision. To complete the chapter, I then provide details of three real-life provisions to indicate how Creative Health practitioners have responded to different contexts with considered and selective promotional voices.

Scientific Voice

Tangible resources, by their very nature, can be readily described and, to some extent, measured. Take, for example, Winnie's commentary on electric cars. Winnie explained that whilst electric cars have much to offer environmentally, the infrastructure means that they are not accessible to poorer individuals. In particular, Winnie described how people living in terrace houses cannot park outside their houses in order to charge their cars, and limitations like these prevent them from staying in touch with the progression of society (Winnie, 2022). Another example that Winnie described was regarding physical resources like timetables. Winnie said that they rely on public transport to get around, but since timetables have become digitalised, they have been forced to purchase a phone that can access the internet. The phone becomes far more expensive to people like Winnie, than the costs of printing the timetable, which Winnie describes as a movement of financial responsibility from service-providers to service-users (Winnie, 2022). Winnie provided many other examples of tangible resources which are becoming more expensive to

DOI: 10.4324/9781003423317-27

access and believes that this creates barriers to living for poorer individuals, which in turn impacts their wellbeing. Because of the tangibility of these resources and the specificity of Winnie's claimed impacts, this could be measured within a study and a value could be attributed to these tangible resources.

This is a traditional way of marketing. However, the values that many Creative Health professionals promote are related to intangible resources, meaning their conceptualisation is particularly subjected to the personal interpretation and resonance of their service-user. Whilst some provisions can be backed by scientific statements of benefits, for many provisions these are either unavailable (due to lack of research or lack of measurement tools) or do not capture the right tone for the provision and their target market. To demonstrate, I reflect on the Gong Bath example presented in the introduction to this book. Within an existing service, a service-provider's gong baths were promoted using the phrasing 'Allow yourself to immerse in the healing vibrations of sound' (Kozera, 2022, para. 1). Below I describe this provision using scientific language. I will then readdress this example using the different techniques discussed throughout this chapter.

> *Gong baths are a type of music therapy which use chime vibrations to encapsulate a person in sound and influence the brainwaves associated with different states of mind.*
>
> *The type of brain wave is defined by the frequency at which it is pulsing. […] Alpha brain waves (8–12 Hz) […] Theta brain waves (3–8 Hz) […] Depending on the activity of brain at a time, particular brain waves will dominate over others (Hima et al., 2020).*

> *Advocates of gong baths claim that they can alter alpha and theta brainwaves, which causes the brain to relax and process the day, leaving users in a calmer state.*
>
> *There is an absence of scientific studies into this area, but theories propose that manipulation of Alpha and Theta brain waves might increase creativity and wellbeing (Boynton, 2001). Small tests have sought to show that increasing alpha brainwaves through music can lead to enhanced memory retention (Makada et al., 2016) but the small sample size of this study calls for extra research in this area. Larger scale studies have obtained user-reports that gong baths help them to achieve 'durable inner peace […] better physical and mental wellbeing, fresh impetus for work, desire for personal growth and other positive effects' (Pesek and Bratina, 2016). Observational studies into comparable music therapies have indicated a reduction in 'tension, anger, fatigue, and depressed mood' along with increased spiritual well-being (Goldsby et al., 2017).*

Storytelling Voice

Within the participant interviews, **intangible resources** were communicated about through creative storytelling, rather than measurements and scientific pathways. For example, Gayle described their emotional response to seeing war planes flying in and out of their base. They demonstrated just how difficult these intangible resources can be to describe, saying, 'I couldn't explain to anybody, and nobody could quite get the moment [...] I can't explain what... it was just a wonder' (Gayle, 2021). How Gayle chose to elicit an emotional response that aligned to their experience, was through describing the story rather than the resource. They used language such as 'it was quite quiet, just a bird singing, and just me cycling along this country lane' which set a visual context, 'I looked up and [...] I thought "come on [Gayle] you're doing a good job"' which demonstrated Gayle's emotional response and thought process, and 'I've never forgotten so long as I live' which demonstrated the scale that this event impacted them (Gayle, 2021).

This peripheral information, elicited via creative storytelling, could not replicate Gayle's experience, but it offered a strong sensation of what it may have been like. This same use of storytelling may find its place within service-providers promotional material. A good example of how storytelling can be brought into promotional communication is via user testimonials and metaphor. To demonstrate the use of these, I return to the example of gong baths using an imagined testimonial (for illustrative purposes only).

Gong Bath, User Testimonial:

> *I came to my first gong bath feeling tired – both physically and mentally-overburdened with work, and angry about what my life had become. After the first session I felt calmer and went home to the best sleep I had experienced in a long time. It felt like an important pause in my, otherwise, busy life and I felt proud that I had given myself that time.*
>
> *Now I attend the sessions monthly and I feel like my sense of meaning is coming back. In the first week after a session, I always feel that my focus and memory as slightly sharper, but more importantly I just carry this beautiful memory of lying there, surrounded by gongs, letting myself drift off into daydreams. Remembering the sessions is obviously not the same as being there, but it does provide me with a sense of calm – almost like a visual (memory) reminder that I am important and that I need to balance my needs with the needs of my work.*

This type of promotion is more personable and allows the promoter to focus on the strengths of their impact to those who enjoy the provision, rather than trying to ascertain whether the service works for everyone and to what degree, via a particular brain-related measurement. For researchers and service-providers who choose to gather testimonials, I advise that prompts are offered, so that the specific details of what service-users enjoy are gathered. Participant accounts which are vaguer (such as, 'I love this service. You should totally go!') help to demonstrate enthusiasm but fail to model for new audiences how they could benefit from the service or why they should consider attending.

Poetic Voice

Another approach to describing intangible resources within my research interviews, was for participants to speak of them poetically. An example of this is Ngoen's description of a culturally informed aspect of their wellbeing as 'that wholesome feeling when you see someone and it just reminds you of good food' (Ngoen, 2022). In another example, Ngoen discussed the act of making jokes, saying that giving people laughter is a valuable source of wellbeing. Being precise in their meaning, Ngoen described 'the intimacy - the courage to go into that person's space' - associated with sharing risky humour (Ngoen, 2022).

Other examples include Winnie's conviction that the atmosphere of a train 'can send a thrill through you, sometimes' (Winnie, 2022) and that there is joy in walking in somebody's company without the expectation or need to talk (Winnie, 2022). A final example, from Kris, described the intangible benefits of yoga:

> everyone's lying down [...] and it gets me so emotional sometimes [...] because when you see bodies just doing nothing... [...] I look around and I just see, like, books [...] If they could write a story, I'd read it.
>
> (Kris, 2021)

These more poetic approaches to value description draw upon embodied notions of joy, visual depictions, and interrelation commentary to simulate the actual experience of an intangible resource. Since these more poetic ways of speaking appeared so often, it is possible that they might be used in promotional material also. But caution much be taken with this tone. Language which verges too far into the abstract or non-descript can have the opposite effect of isolating an individual, particularly where access needs may be present (e.g., neurodivergent people who manage their anxiety and aid their social modelling via clear, pragmatic descriptions of what they can expect). Moreover, since poetic communication risks being particularly personal in its form and interpretation, service-providers may choose to supplement it with language that is more traditionally professional in tone.

An example of how poetic voice might be applied to gong baths is:

> *Imagine getting into a bath, turning on the tap and hearing it pour with deep radiating sounds. This is the concept of a gong bath – a music*

sensation that enwraps its listeners in a healing blanket of vibration. Swap those soapy bubbles for a deep cleanse of all the negative emotions bubbling up inside of you. These warm penetrating sounds will help you to elicit a sense of calm and will position you in a state of mind which is focused and able to reflect. The perfect treat for all the shower lovers out there!

In this example, you will note that romanticised language is coupled with clear expected outcomes. The specifics of the intended benefits help to invite the audience into the more abstract world of poetics, appropriately preparing them for the transition into the artistic space of gong baths.

Another important note about these more expressive forms of promotion, is that whilst they can be very attractive to service-users, they may lack the clarity and measurability that investors desire. In this case, the explicit use of the word 'intangible resources' may be an important distinction to make, early within the bidding process, particularly when followed by a rationale of why this type of resource should not be measured. Service-providers can then fall back on other clear descriptors, identified throughout this framework, to clarify the things they can communicate using market-friendly language, and advocate for an adaptable expression of values.

Real-World Examples from the Field of Creative Health

In my first example from real-life Creative Health contexts, I will be discussing a resource I created for the National Centre for Creative health, entitled *Creative Health a Glance* (Hearst, 2024). In this resource, my primary target audience was senior leaders within Integrated Care Boards. Often coming from clinical backgrounds, I wanted the tone of my promotion to represent what they were used to. This demanded reference to clear and rigorous statistics. To aid this, I partnered with Library and Knowledge Services at Midlands Partnership University NHS Foundation Trust, whereby librarians are available to support NHS staff in creating scoping reviews. Emma George, the librarian who collected most of the statistics, searched through academic databases using key-terms that I provided and looked out for sources that met the criteria I outlined. One of these criteria was that I was looking for quantitative data over qualitative, in the first instance, and that this data should signal the financial or health savings that are made possible through a provision. Another criterion was that the health conditions featured should be one of those that appear in the NHS's Core20PLUS5 strategy, the government's Major Conditions Strategy, or be related to Frailty and Falls (one of the leading causes of hospital admissions in the UK). By focusing on these three areas of priority for the health systems, I was able to demonstrate where Creative Health might play a role in addressing the health conditions that are putting the most strain on the NHS. By focusing my language on financial savings, value for money, and increasing capacity, I was able to talk to leaders on their own terms and quickly convert Creative Health sceptics into intrigued advocates and pioneers.

Around a similar time to the publication of my resource, a film by Samantha Moore (*Visible Mending*, 2023) was touring around film festivals across the UK. The film, Visible Mending, is a BAFTA Nominated short Documentary film, demonstrating 'the role knitting plays in many peoples' lives; helping them face adversity, calm anxiety, and make crucial social connections' (British Council, 2024) This film captured the real-life stories of people in a Shropshire knitting group and coupled the voice-overs with knitted animal characters, who creatively visualised the content of discussions. The stop-motion animation was developed by a team in Birmingham, called Second Home Studios, who capture the imaginations of the audience through unexpected juxtapositions and a heart-warming narrative development. This film is an expert representation of what is possible within the narrative promotion space, using both language and visuals to move an audience.

Finally, in a co-production project I developed for the National Centre for Creative Health, in collaboration with the National Arts in Hospitals Network and University Hospitals of Derby and Burton NHS Trust, Hospital Arts Managers from across the Midlands were invited to join artists and hospital staff to explore the theme of workforce wellbeing. In this session, we wanted to remove the NHS hierarchies which can stunt safe and equitable expression. Moreover, we wanted to ensure that participants were left feeling light and hopeful, rather than worn out from the exploration of difficult mental health stories. The way that we achieved both of these aims was by inviting an artistic facilitator to conduct a range of poetry-based exercises. The poet, Beth Calverley, used bright visual prompts and spacial exploration among her activities, to harness a sense of intrigue and play within the participants. Poems were developed collectively using a verbatim poetry approach. In one activity, this involved participants responding to a range of prompts around the room with short words or sentences. An example of one of these prompts was 'wellbeing feels like...' (*Derby Workforce Wellbeing Huddle*, 2024). Answers from each were then selected at random by the participants – one per prompt – and collated into a collective poem. In another activity, Beth asked us to respond to visual prompts with creative ideas. During the sharing of these ideas, she scribed some of the pertinent quotes from people in the room. At the end of the discussion, Beth read this collection of quotes back, using a poetic tone, demonstrating to us another way of developing collaborative verbatim poetry. This creative approach to discussing wellbeing allowed the group to discuss the theme on new terms and engage their creative problem-solving skills. This supported the collaborative nature of the initiative, whilst still collecting quality outputs. We followed the poetry session with a Theory of Change development session, allowing participants to turn ideas into meaningful action.

Final Thoughts...

Tone of voice can, undoubtedly, be a highly personal preference. It is no surprise, then, that we often feel compelled to discuss our work in a way that resonates strongly to us, since this is easier for us to model the emotional reaction to what we have said. But others are not like us. Even if they are moved on an emotional level, they may not be able to interact with our work in the way that we intend – say commissioners – if we do not provide them with the information and framing that they need. It is my hope that by discussing three possible tones in this chapter, Creative Health practitioners will we inspired to explore tone in their own promotional contexts and feel confident to adapt information to different target audiences. These three voices are not intended to be exhaustive, so I invite you to think outside the box and add to this frame with your own knowledge of tone. However, the three voices outlined here are those that were most prominent in the stories of my research participants – ordinary members of the public – pointing to familiar and effective ways of communicating, which carry recognisable patterns of application.

References

Boynton, T. (2001) Applied research using alpha/theta training for enhancing creativity and well-being. *Journal of Neurotherapy*, 5(1–2), pp. 5–18.

British Council (2024) *Visible Mending*. London: British Council, Online.

Derby Workforce Wellbeing Huddle. (2024) [Poetry on film] Directed by *Derby Workforce Wellbeing Huddle*. The National Centre for Creative Health.

Gayle (2021) Interview with Jane Hearst.

Goldsby, T.L. et al. (2017) Effects of singing bowl sound meditation on mood, tension, and well-being: An observational study. *Journal of Evidence-Based Complementary & Alternative Medicine*, 22(3), pp. 401–406.

Hearst, J. (2024) *Creative Health at a Glance: Core20PLUS5, Major Conditions, & Falls Prevention*. Nottingham: The National Centre for Creative Health.

Hima, C.S. et al. (2020) A review on brainwave therapy. *World Journal of Pharmaceutical Sciences*, 8(11), pp. 59–66.

Kozera, K. (2022) *Yoga & Sound*. [Online] Surya Yoga Sound. Available at: https://www.instagram.com/p/Cg1WEi1s8E4/ [Accessed 01/10/2022].

Kris (2021) Interview with Jane Hearst.

Makada, T. et al. (2016) Enhancing Memory Retention by Increasing Alpha and Decreasing Beta Brainwaves using Music. In: *Proceedings of the 9th ACM International Conference on PErvasive Technologies Related to Assistive Environments. PETRA '16: 9th ACM International Conference on PErvasive Technologies Related to Assistive Environments*. Corfu Island Greece: ACM, pp. 1–4.

Ngoen (2022) Interview with Jane Hearst.

Pesek, A. and Bratina, T. (2016) Gong and its therapeutic meaning. *Musicological Annual*, 52(2), pp. 137–161.

Visible Mending. (2023) [Non-fiction animation] Directed by Directed by Samantha Moore. London: British Council. Available at: https://vimeo.com/827066711 [Accessed: 27/10/2024].

Winnie (2022) Interview with Jane Hearst.

Conclusion

Reflections on the Book

This book has covered three distinct areas of contribution to the field of Creative Health. The first is a strategic analysis of the market, looking at how our capitalist economy shapes decisions about healthcare, how the philosophies and practises of traditional healthcare systems affect the integration of Creative Health, and how our current rhetoric around Creative Health supports or dismantles power relations. The second is a person-centred view of market research, looking at how a pragmatist epistemological framework improves the chances of research impacting provisions in the market, how critical psychology illuminates the negotiation that takes place between a service-user and the market, and how narrative development activities are an effective way of engaging service-users in market-related research projects. Finally, the Creative Health Communication Framework offers a practical tool for Creative Health researchers and practitioners working in mental health and wellbeing, supporting better communication about what threats they are supporting, how they are supporting the service-user, and the wider context of their provision.

Combined, these areas of contribution demonstrate the importance of considering market forces during the design, implementation, and communication about Creative Health services. Readers can use the knowledge throughout these pages to improve the compatibility of their services to service-users, communicate the overall value of their service to commissioners, and improve their chances of market success.

One of the transformative aspects of the Creative Health Communication Framework is that it centres members of the public and their preferred communication styles in its development. Thanks to this, I have developed a framework that best represents how service-users like to talk about their mental health and wellbeing, making the field more inclusive, whilst still appealing to the market concerns of healthcare commissioners.

DOI: 10.4324/9781003423317-28

The Potential Impact of the Creative Health Communication Framework

This framework has the capacity to change current practises in the mental health and wellbeing sectors, as it allows us to map a wide variety of services and understand their unique offering. This, therefore, could support senior mental health managers and social prescribers in allocating more compatible services to users and reducing waiting list via the lower reliance on clinical provisions.

The specific industry challenge that this framework addresses is the inadequate communication of what wellbeing is being supported via services and how. The framework effectively isolates four distinct areas of differentiation in the type of threat to wellbeing that is being supported, four more distinctions in how the service-provider will respond to these threats, and four important contextual factors. These factors, combined, allow service-providers to be explicitly clear in what distinguishes them from other provisions – helping to inspire trust in their users and make their value clear to commissioners.

I envision practitioners applying this framework in the development of research proposals, in discussion with healthcare commissioners, during cultural bid-writing, on social prescribing platforms, in social media promotions, and in direct communication with those that they support. Healthcare leaders can also use this to shape the type of information they gather in application forms, the things they measure in evidence projects, and the way they map services over their local jurisdiction.

Future Directions for This Work

When I first conceived of a Creative Health Communication Framework, one of the key outcomes that I wanted to enable was the mapping of Creative Health provisions at a local scale. How I envisaged this taking place was through the selection of one or two frames – such as the wellbeing orientations – and applying them to the intended outcomes of local artists. This would lead to distinct bubbles of activity – in this case seven subsections of wellbeing that are being supported – which could be visualised across a city or region, demonstrating where there are gaps in the market. This type of information can be compared to data that records the prevalence of needs for the local population, allowing health leaders to effectively respond to gaps in the market and over saturation of provisions, with reallocation of financial and in-kind resources.

Since completing the Creative Health Communication Framework, I have received interest from stakeholders in the field of social prescribing to integrate the frames into their work. Potential developments in this area include the development of training on the use of the framework for Social

Prescribers/Link Workers. Another option is incorporating the framework into social prescribing case management systems. This would make it easier for busy GPs to interact with social prescribing approaches, without needing to invest extensive time in learning about local provisions. The system would direct questions to primary care patients and, in response to their preferences, identify the most compatible local services based on mental health needs (rather than, or in addition to, artform preference). This would increase the confidence of GPs and Social Prescribers in linking patients to quality provisions, whilst avoiding biases. Moreover, these categorisations would enable tracking of progress, if desired, which, in turn, supports the development of more evidence in the Creative Health field.

Elsewhere, stakeholders from Mental Health Transformation teams, ICBs, PCNs, and public health teams have expressed an interest in the Creative Health Communication Framework. Whilst we have yet to identify specific means of incorporating this into their work, their interest and advocacy signals an exciting opportunity to integrate more person-centred healthcare across the systems. Collectively, their efforts could make a considerable impact on the quality, diversity, and compatibility of mental health provisions available to members of the public.

One particular area of application that links to this would be the use of the framework within Arts Collectives. These groups – such as Number 11 Arts, who are spread across Birmingham City – are increasingly accessed by healthcare teams – like the public health team in Birmingham – to engage artists in paid health delivery work. The framework would help them to map what the strengths are of different artists in their network, which, in turn, would enable a fair and appropriate distribute of work, moving away from discriminatory practices such as the prioritisation of large organisations over local knowledge experts.

As artistic commissioners – such as Arts Council England – integrate Creative Health streams into their work, there is the opportunity to trial the use of the framework in the evaluation of funding bids. Similar initiatives may be of use to healthcare organisations, during their procurement procedures, or for cross-disciplinary network facilitators, such as Cultural Compacts.

Additionally, the gamification of the Creative Health Communication Framework would allow for a fun and interactive method of increasing mental health literacy and awareness in the general population. For example, this might entail players interacting with Non-Playable Characters (NPCs), responding to visible character stats, with the goal of improving the wellbeing of both NPCs and themselves.

Thinking more widely, I hope that one day, this framework will not only be used in the field of Creative Health, as it has potential to impact the mental health and wellbeing industries at large. Moreover, whilst this framework has focused on mental health and wellbeing, there is still space to develop comparable frameworks for other aspects of our health. One particular example which comes to mind is a framework for how Creative Health can respond to 'wicked issues' – complex and persistent health issues that are difficult to define, lack a clear solution, and are often interconnected with other problems.

Final Visionary Note

This book has attempted to contribute not only to the field of Creative Health but also to the field of mental health and wellbeing more broadly. I believe that the application of this framework can lead towards more compassionate and person-centred healthcare, making Creative Health leaders pioneers in the field. This was made possible through my consideration of the market and thanks to my pragmatic, collaborative approach to design. I hope that more and more healthcare leaders can apply similar values to their own work, thereby improving the growth and quality of our healthcare innovation.

The Creative Health Communication Framework is emergent. It was created in response to a particular type of market and with service-users who communicate about mental health and wellbeing in a way that reflects the common communication style at that moment in time. The success of the framework will rely on its ongoing innovation, responding to market developments and increased mental health literacy. More work with targeted demographics will help us to understand the degree to which the framework can contribute towards agendas, such as decolonisation and the disenfranchisement of minoritised groups, supporting important reductions in health inequalities.

Ultimately, the impact gained from this framework and the information explored in this book will be dependent on you, the readers, and your networks. You have the power to improve the quality and visibility of Creative Health provisions. Together, we can help Creative Health to thrive across our communities.

Index

Pages in *italics* refer to figures.

For Product Safety Concerns and Information please contact our EU representative GPSR@taylorandfrancis.com Taylor & Francis Verlag GmbH, Kaufingerstraße 24, 80331 München, Germany

Batch number: 10406157

Printed by Printforce, the Netherlands